Some comments from people whc  ok:

"I have used these (allergy and tolerar.   ,,,, methods with a number of people. Their most common response is, 'It's a miracle!'"
David Rowland, Ph.D., R.N.C., President, Nutritional Consultants Organization of Canada

"I wish I had been able to learn this years ago. To think of all the people who could have been really helped."
V.W., Austria

"Nothing else helped, but my daughter is finally well."
N.L., France

"Your technique has been so valuable. We use it constantly."
G.F., Denmark

"It's amazing!"
B.K., New York

"Your method has changed my life."
M.E., England

"It really works. I use it all the time."
C.P., California

"This technique has changed how I practice medicine."
A.K., Germany

"I didn't believe it until I tried it. Even though I now know it works, I still can't believe it!"
C.C., Switzerland

Cure Your Own Allergies

IN MINUTES

Jimmy Scott, Ph.D.

with Kathleen Goss, M.A.

Illustrations by Claudia Wagar

Health Kinesiology Publications

San Francisco 1988

The following are trademarks of The Health Kinesiology Institute

Health Kinesiology™
Balancing Tap™
Allergy Tap™
Tolerance Tap™
Energy Flow Balancing™
HKPapers™
Symbiotic Energy Transformation™ (SET™)

No part of this book may be copied, reproduced, or transmitted in any form or by any means, electronic or mechanical, including but not limited to photocopying, photography, recording, or by any information storage and retrieval system, without prior agreement and written permission from the publisher. Excepted are brief quotations when included in a review.

Copyright © 1988 by Jimmy Scott, Ph.D. All rights reserved.

Manufactured in the United States of America

Library of Congress Cataloging-in-Publication Data:
Scott, Jimmy, 1938-
        Cure your own allergies in minutes / Jimmy Scott with
Kathleen Goss; illustrations by Claudia Ricketts Wagar
            xvi+224p.   15 x 20 cm.
            Includes index.
            ISBN 0-945509-01-4 : $14.95
            1. Allergy.   2. Self-Care, Health.   3. Kinesiology.   I. Goss,
Kathleen. II. Title.
        RC585.S38 1988
        616.97--dc 19   88-3114
                                                                   CIP

Health Kinesiology Publications
1032 Irving Street, Suite 340
San Francisco, Ca 94122
(415) 566-4611

Other books by Jimmy Scott, Ph.D.

Energy, Allergy, and Your Health. Second edition.
 A companion to *Cure Your Own Allergies in Minutes.*
 In preparation.

Relieve Your Own Emotional Distress and Phobias in Minutes.
 In preparation.

Dr. Scott's High-Calorie Weight Control Diet (and Program for Good Health).
 In preparation.

Improve Your Own Intellectual Functioning and Creativity in Minutes.
 In preparation.

Emotions Training.
 In preparation.

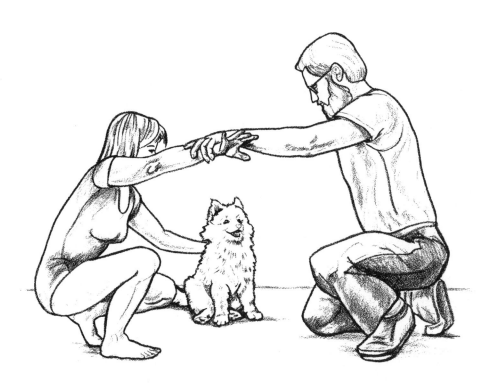

Surrogate Testing Rimsky. See Chapter 5.

Acknowledgments

Kathleen Goss, who, with amazing ease, manages to convert my ideas and procedures into organized prose. Except for Kathy's work this book would have been finished about five years later. She has been perfect to work with.

Claudia Wagar, for being a talented and patient artist.

Lydia Temoshok, Ken Wagar, and Rimsky-Korsakov VI, for being such wonderful models for the artist.

The Graphic Eye, of Berkeley, Ca., and especially Suellen Ehnebuske, for the cover design and for transforming stacks of drawings, piles of papers, and numerous half-formed ideas, into a *real* book!

Christina Taccone, for the photograph of the author with Rimsky, his favorite Samoyed (on the back cover).

Most of all I thank those hundreds of clients and friends without whom I could not have learned the things I write about.

Cure your Own Allergies in Minutes is also published as:

Vaincre ses Allergies en Quelques Minutes

> Guy Saint-Jean Éditeur Inc.
> 674, Place Publique, bureau 200
> Laval Québec Canada
> H7X 1G1
> (514) 332-5860

Allergiefrei—eine Sache von Minuten

> Verlag für Angewandte Kinesiologie
> Zasiusstraße 67
> D-7800 Freiburg
> West Germany
> 07 61 / 7 27 29

Bevrijd Jezelf van Je Allergie in een Handomdraai

> Ankh-Hermes
> Uitgeverij ANKH-HERMES bv
> Smyrnastraat 5
> NL-7413 BA Deventer
> Holland
> 05700-33355

Other languages forthcoming

Contents

Disclaimer

We believe that you, as an individual, are responsible for your own health and that you cannot give up this responsibility to others. The role of health professionals is to work with the individual to determine the best possible set of strategies for restoring and maintaining health in each case. Thus a wide range of appropriately qualified professionals may be able to provide assistance in achieving this goal.

In the course of following the instructions in this book, you may be exposed to substances to which you are highly reactive. If you know or suspect that you have severe sensitivities to certain substances, use extreme caution in handling them. If in any doubt about how to deal with such substances, consult a properly qualified professional.

The results of the testing techniques described herein may lead you to consider eliminating or reducing the dosages of medicines you are currently taking, or making other changes in your consumption of foods and other substances. Before making any changes in your present medicines, you may wish to consult with the responsible health professional; together you will be able to work out an appropriate way to make these changes. Your need for most drugs will diminish as you get healthier.

If your health professional disagrees with the ideas in this book, feel free to seek a second or third opinion. Since you are completely responsible for your own health, you are free to consult anyone you choose, and then to make your own decision. Chapter 10 provides some suggestions about how to locate qualified health professionals who will be able to help you to understand and apply the techniques we describe herein.

The methods and ideas described in this book are not orthodox. Consequently, orthodox practitioners may criticize or "put down" these procedures, or even *you* for considering them. However, the final judge is still you. If the procedures work for you, then their value is proven regardless of the opinion of some "authority" who does not understand them. Your own health improvement will be more convincing than any words.

The purpose of this book is not to diagnose or prescribe, nor to teach you to do so. Since these procedures are so new they cannot be considered to be proven scientifically to be valid or even useful. You must use these methods at your own risk. However, the extensive experience of the author, and many others he has trained, has not yet revealed any untoward reaction, with the possible exception of occasional slight muscle soreness due to excessive muscle testing. The author believes these procedures to be valid and useful, or else this book would not have been written.

Preface

YOU ARE PROBABLY ALLERGIC!

Most likely you have allergies. You may not think of yourself as an allergic type of person because you don't have common allergic symptoms such as rash, runny nose, or difficulty breathing. But if you have any physical or psychological problems at all, chances are that at least some of them are related to allergies to foods or environmental substances. Furthermore, many times allergic problems are not recognized or are actually hidden. In recent years a very wide range of symptoms have been found to be partly due, at least sometimes, to allergy.

In the past, it was not very easy to determine whether a person's symptoms were due to allergy. Skin testing and other commonly employed methods tend to be expensive, time consuming, and unreliable.[a] Even if you or your doctor suspected you had an allergy, it might be difficult to prove it, or to determine to what substance you were allergic.

Now, using the information in this book, you can find out for yourself, in your own home, whether you, your family members, or friends have allergies. A simple testing method, based on a new concept of allergy as a disturbance of the body's energy, makes it possible for anyone, working with a friend, to test for allergies to virtually any substance. Not only that, using the techniques in this book, you can also *eliminate* your allergies in about 90 percent of cases!

---

[a] It was proven in the 1930s that skin testing was unreliable for the determination of food allergies.

How These Methods Were Developed

I have been working with nutrition and allergy for more than ten years. In my practice I have observed over and over again that allergies can produce just about any kind of symptom imaginable, and that when allergic problems are eliminated many previously "incurable" conditions simply go away. Several years ago, I began developing new energy procedures to deal with the psychological factors that affect people's health. The allergy correction procedures described in this book were an outgrowth of that work. I discovered that the stage is set for most allergic problems very early in life, when psychological issues begin to interfere with the body's energy flow. Since a proper flow of energy is required to regulate many bodily functions, a disturbance in the energy flow can cause regulation to fail, and problems such as allergies begin to appear.

Once energy disturbances have set the stage for allergies, many other factors can contribute to the problem. Nutritional deficiencies, lack of exercise, toxicity, psychological stresses—all add to the burden on your body and further disturb its energy flow. Optimal health depends on proper attention to all these factors; but by directly working to rebalance the body's energy we can make it easier for these other functions to be restored to normal.[b]

In my early allergy work, I relied on methods such as fasting, mono food testing (eating one food at a time), and pulse testing to determine if a person was allergic to various substances.[c] These techniques are generally relatively cumbersome, uncomfortable, and slow, but they were the best available at the time. Later, applying the energy approach to allergy, I began to use a set of muscle testing techniques which proved to be much

---

[b] The role of nutritional deficiencies and other factors in the development of allergies is discussed in my book *Energy, Allergy, and Your Health*.

[c] By fasting and then reintroducing foods, one by one, we are able to observe possible allergic reactions. Pulse testing is a technique introduced by Dr. Arthur Coca, who observed that the pulse rate increases after eating a food to which one is allergic.

more sensitive and reliable. Suddenly, all the old allergy testing methods were obsolete.

For several years I used muscle testing techniques to identify people's allergies, and we would then work to correct them through avoidance of the allergic substances, proper diet, and nutritional supplementation. This procedure was effective but time consuming, often taking six months to a year or more. Then, in 1982, I discovered and began to develop new energy techniques for *correcting* allergies, as well as identifying them. This procedure is now highly developed and is included, along with several other techniques, in a comprehensive system I call *Health Kinesiology*. Using techniques such as these, I have usually been able to eliminate people's allergies during a single office visit, as opposed to the long and often uncomfortable months of dietary intervention that had been my principal approach in the past.

Health Kinesiology requires extensive knowledge of many energy reflex points in the body, and cannot be done by an untrained person. However, more recently I have discovered that in a very high percentage of cases a much shorter and simpler set of techniques, not requiring professional training, is sufficient to eliminate most allergies. This *Allergy Tap* technique is the quick method of allergy correction described in this book. It is effective in about 90 percent of cases. A simple test, also described in this book, enables you to determine whether the Allergy Tap will work to eliminate an allergy to a specific substance in a specific person.

How to Use This Book

You will find the energy techniques easiest and most reliable to use if you understand the principles on which they are based. For this reason, Chapters 1-4 provide explanations of the body's energy system and the energy concept of allergy, along with the specific procedures for energy balancing, muscle testing, allergy testing, allergy energy balancing, tolerance testing, and tolerance energy balancing. Complete descriptions of all these procedures are brought together in Appendix A. You are encouraged to try the procedures as you encounter them in reading through the text, but once you have read the complete text it will be more convenient to refer to the descriptions of the procedures in Appendix A. When you become thoroughly familiar with the procedures, you will only need to refer to the short summaries and flowcharts in Appendix B to jog your memory.

A special feature of this book is the Illustrations section. All illustrations referred to in the text are collected here, just before the Appendices. Dark bars along the edges of the pages make it easy to find this section for quick reference.

What to Expect

It is common in many health practices today to engage in what we call "blaming the victim"—that is, to assume that the sufferer from illness is somehow responsible for the symptoms he or she is experiencing. You are *not* to blame for your allergies. The stage was set for your allergic problems early in your life, often by psychological processes beyond your control. But now, with these energy techniques at your disposal, you *can* be responsible for *eliminating* your allergies. It may not be your fault that you are suffering from your symptoms, but it is your fault if you don't do something to correct them! Remember, however, that the actual healing of the body's tissues lags behind the energy correction procedures; do not expect "miracles" to occur overnight. Moreover, best results are obtained when the energy correction procedures are accompanied by a proper nutritional support program, including both diet changes and nutritional supplements.

We humans are all very different. The importance of allergies varies greatly from one person to another. For some people, the allergy correction procedures described in this book will produce dramatic changes. For others, they will produce virtually no obvious changes. For everyone, however, this book provides an opportunity to experience how the body's energy works, and to learn how to use the inner wisdom of our own bodies to determine what they need. I am sure you will find the experience educational and exciting.

To all those people who

believe that only they

themselves can be responsible

for their own well-being and

ultimate happiness

HOW TO CURE

YOUR OWN

ALLERGIES

1

Do You Have Allergies?

Many people, perhaps yourself included, suffer from distressing physical or mental symptoms for which they have not been able to obtain relief. Have you ever gone to a medical doctor, only to be told your problem is all in your imagination? Or have you been told you have a certain disease, and yet the prescribed treatment does nothing to help you?

In many such cases the real problem is allergy. In my nutritional and health counseling practice, I have seen time and time again that when an underlying allergic problem is identified and eliminated, many illnesses simply go away (assuming adequate nutrition has been provided also).

Most health care professionals do not think to look for allergy in difficult cases, and even if they do, they may not use methods adequate to analyze the problem. Thus, for a number of reasons, many of us suffer from unrecognized, "hidden" allergies.

For a long time, the idea of allergy was confined to a small group of obvious symptoms such as runny nose, red eyes, sneezing, or skin rash. Today, health professionals recognize that a much wider range of problems may sometimes be due to allergy, including digestive problems, headaches, muscle aches and pains, arthritis, poor blood sugar control, addictions, and psychological and behavioral problems, among many others.

If allergy is suspected in such cases, a variety of tests may be used to try to identify the substances to which the individual is allergic. Allergy specialist physicians often use skin testing, while clinical ecologists use sublingual testing (placing a tiny amount of the suspect substance under the person's tongue), or other more appropriate tests. Cytotoxic testing is a new form of allergy testing which looks for reactions in the white blood cells under a microscope when they are exposed to the substance in question.

Unfortunately, in my experience, most of these forms of allergy testing are not sufficiently accurate to identify many allergies, especially those which are hidden. This book will introduce you to a new set of tools to identify allergies which might not show up on conventional testing. Later in this chapter you will learn how to test yourself for allergies, using a simple method that you can do with a friend.

Why Are Allergies Hidden?

There are three main reasons why allergies may be hidden. First, the symptoms may be masked by the mucus which the body produces to protect itself against the substances to which it is allergic. Secondly, allergic symptoms may not be directly observable—they may not be the kinds of symptoms that would show up on allergy testing, or they may be changes in parts of the body that can't be observed directly, such as the early changes in a joint capsule which ultimately lead to arthritis. A third reason why allergies may be hidden is that the symptoms may not be recognized as allergic. It may surprise you, for example, that high blood pressure often has an allergic basis. Muscle tension is another common problem that can be allergic in origin, as can many mental and behavioral problems including hyperactivity and learning disabilities in children.[1]

---

[1] See my book *Energy, Allergy, and Your Health* for more information about hidden allergies.

Review Your Symptoms

Now let's repeat our initial question. Do you have any symptoms for which you have been unable to obtain help? This book will show you how you can determine if these problems are related to allergy.

Before going any further, look at the checklist of possible allergy symptoms in Table 1. After you have used this book to correct your allergic problems, you can go back to this checklist sometime in the future and see if the symptoms you have checked have gone away, or even if any new symptoms have developed. You will probably be surprised to see how many of your everyday complaints, as well as more serious problems, go away when your allergy problems are resolved. Remember, however, that only about 90% of all allergies can be corrected with this method.

* * *

A tremendous variety of symptoms is recognized today as caused by allergy. The following list is representative of the range of problems that are known or suspected to indicate allergies, in at least some cases. Remember, too, that most symptoms can be produced by a variety of causes.

Before reading further in this book, write today's date in the first column. For each symptom indicate in the adjacent space in column 1 the degree to which you are experiencing that symptom, right now, according to the scale. Feel free to make any additions to the list you need. At the end of the checklist, record the total number of points for today's date.

Later, after you have used the allergy correction techniques described in this book, review the checklist again, perhaps three months and six months from now. Be sure to put the new date in the next column. Continue to evaluate your symptoms periodically to see how you are progressing. (Before filling out this checklist, you may want to make photocopies of it, so that you can use it many times to monitor your own symptoms, and those of other family members, over time.)

In Appendix G is an anonymous report form for you to use to send to the author a summary of your experiences with these methods. These results will be tabulated for research purposes.

TABLE 1

CHECKLIST OF ALLERGIC SYMPTOMS

0 = none   1 = mild   2 = moderate   3 = severe

	Degree of symptom (0-3)			
	Date:	Date:	Date:	Date:
	___	___	___	___

GASTROINTESTINAL

Inflamed, sore lips	___	___	___	___
Canker sores	___	___	___	___
"Geographic" tongue (alternating bald and furry patches)	___	___	___	___
Excessive salivation	___	___	___	___
Itching of roof of mouth	___	___	___	___
Air swallowing	___	___	___	___
Nausea	___	___	___	___
Vomiting	___	___	___	___
Heartburn	___	___	___	___
Indigestion	___	___	___	___
Bloating	___	___	___	___
Belching	___	___	___	___
Passing gas	___	___	___	___
Repeating a taste	___	___	___	___
Nervous stomach	___	___	___	___
Abdominal pain	___	___	___	___
Ulcer	___	___	___	___
Cramps	___	___	___	___
Diarrhea	___	___	___	___
Constipation	___	___	___	___
Blood or mucus in stool	___	___	___	___
Anal itching	___	___	___	___

SKIN
  Hives or welts
  Dermatitis (eczema)
  Adult acne
  Itching
  Burning
  Flushing
  Pallor
  Excessive sweating

GENERAL APPEARANCE
  Pale and sallow appearance
  Swollen face
  Enlarged lymph glands
  Excess weight
  Excess thinness

RESPIRATORY
  Runny nose
  Itching nose
  Nasal congestion
  Nasal polyps
  Sneezing
  Postnasal discharge
  Nosebleed
  Hay fever
  Laryngitis
  Frequent clearing of throat
  Cough or wheeze
  Night cough
  Coughing up phlegm
  Asthma
  Difficulty breathing
  Bronchitis
  Shortness of breath
  Emphysema

CARDIOVASCULAR
  Rapid heart beat
  Palpitations
  Skipped heart beats
  Chest pain
  Ankle or calf swelling
  Fainting spells
  Flushing
  Chills
  Hot flashes
  Night sweats
  High blood pressure
  Low blood pressure

MUSCULOSKELETAL
  Muscle spasm
  Muscle pain
  Muscle cramps
  Muscle weakness
  Neck pain
  Stiff neck
  Arthritis: joint pain, swelling,
    stiffness
  Rheumatism
  Backache

MISCELLANEOUS CONDITIONS
  Anemia
  Addictions (alcohol, drugs, foods)
  Tiredness
  Uterine fibroids
  Fibrocystic breast disease
  Cancer
  Autoimmune diseases

URINARY AND GENITAL
  Frequent urination
  Painful urination
  Burning on urination
  Urinating at night
  Enuresis (poor bladder control,
    bed wetting)
  Urgency to urinate
  Blood in urine
  Incomplete emptying of bladder
  Frequent urinary infections
  Genital itching or pain

EYES
  Eye pain
  Itching
  Photophobia (sensitivity to light)
  Blurred vision
  Refractive changes
  Watering
  Allergic black eyes
  Puffy lids
  Red, bloodshot eyes
  Bags or dark circles under eyes
  Cataract
  Inflammation of iris or cornea

EARS
  Fluid in the ears
  Earache
  Ringing in ears
  Vertigo
  Hearing loss
  Excessive ear wax
  Ear popping
  Flushed, red ear lobes

NERVOUS SYSTEM AND BEHAVIORAL

Headache				
Numbness and tingling				
Restlessness				
Nervousness				
Jitteriness				
Tremor				
Irritability				
Insomnia				
Convulsions				
Anxiety				
Fear or panic reactions				
Confusion				
Clumsiness, poor coordination				
Feelings of apartness, "spaciness"				
Floating sensation				
Amnesia				
Memory problems				
Inability to concentrate				
Learning disorders				
Minimal brain dysfunction				
Hyperactivity				
Behavioral problems				
Inappropriate emotional outbursts				
Uncontrolled anger				
Tension-fatigue syndrome				
Depression				
Personality changes				
Paranoia				
Hallucinations				
Total Points:				

(This Table *may* be copied for your personal use.)

How to Test for Allergies

Now that you have seen that a wide range of problems can be due to allergy, you may be wondering whether any of your own symptoms are allergic in origin. Or, like many people, you may already know that you are allergic to a certain food or other substance. We are now going to describe a set of simple procedures for allergy testing that don't involve visits to doctors' offices, giving blood samples, long waits for test results, or large fees. Before proceeding any further in this book, you can stop right now and learn how to use muscle testing techniques to see whether you are allergic to a specific substance. If you already suspect or know that you are allergic to something, you can use a sample of that substance for the test. If you are not aware of any specific allergies, try the test with one of the more common allergic substances. For example, the most common allergic foods are dairy products and wheat family grains, so any wheat-flour or dairy food would be a good test substance to begin with.

MUSCLE TESTING

Many of the concepts and procedures described in this chapter may seem strange and unfamiliar to you. Before explaining the principles on which muscle testing is based, we would like for you to experience muscle testing directly. As you become familiar with the way it works in practice, the underlying theory will begin to make more sense to you.

The allergy testing procedures described in this book are based on the results of muscle testing. For the sake of convenience, the muscle usually used is one in the upper arm (deltoid muscle). The muscle testing procedure we will describe requires two people. The person administering the test is called the Tester, and the person whose arm is being tested is called the Subject.

Balancing Tap

In order for muscle testing to work as accurately as possible, it is a good idea for both the Tester and the Subject to have their bodies "energy balanced" by performing a simple procedure. We will describe this procedure as the Tester performs it on the Subject; you can then reverse roles, or each person can do it on his or her own.

At the point where your collarbone meets your breastbone, or sternum, you will find a *V* shape at the base of your neck. The Energy Balancing Spot you will be working with is located about 2 inches below this *V*. You will probably feel a small bump on the bone here, at the point where the second ribs attach to the sternum (see Illustration 1 in Illustrations section). Now imagine a circle 3 inches in diameter (or 1-1/2 inches in radius), centering around this Energy Balancing Spot. Facing the Subject, the Tester taps around this circle several times, in a counterclockwise direction, for about 30 seconds (possibly 100 taps), using one or two fingers. Tap firmly but gently, and remember that fingernails can hurt. Ask the other person to let you know if you are tapping too hard; you should be tapping about as hard as you can tap an eggshell without breaking it. You may each tap yourselves, instead of tapping one another.

Muscle Testing

After the energy balancing process is completed, you are ready to go on to muscle testing itself. First try muscle testing in a standing position. The Subject stands, relaxed, with the feet slightly apart, comfortable and balanced. The Subject then holds out one arm, either the left or the right, with the palm facing down. The arm is held about 45 degrees off to the side and about 45 degrees up, as shown in Illustration 2A. You don't have to get the position of the arm exactly correct, but it's a good idea to become accustomed to performing muscle testing in a consistent position, so that you can become familiar with how the muscles feel when they are being tested.

Now the Tester stands facing the Subject and places one hand on one of the Subject's shoulders (for balance), and the other on the Subject's opposite forearm, slightly above the wrist, so that the Tester can press down on the extended arm. The Subject should hold the elbow straight. The Tester can press with the palm, or with all four fingers, or may only need to use one or two fingers, depending on the Subject's strength (see Illustrations 3A and 3B). The Tester says, "Hold," and waits for a moment to allow the Subject to get set holding the arm in position. Then the Tester presses down on the Subject's arm, with a smooth and steady increase in pressure, for about 2-4 seconds, exerting a maximum of about 8-10 pounds of pressure. (You may want to try pressing down on a bathroom scale to get a feel for how much pressure you need.) If this *indicator muscle* is strong the Subject will be able to keep the arm raised against this pressure. If the muscle is weak, the Subject's arm will give way (see Illustration 2B). This is known as testing the indicator muscle *in the clear*. If the muscle tests weak in the clear, redo the Energy Balancing Procedure above before going on with any further testing. If this doesn't work, try the Special Balancing Procedure which is described below and in Appendix A. If that doesn't work, perhaps you are pressing too hard, overpowering the muscle rather than testing it. Try practicing with another person, or use less pressure. Go back over the instructions carefully, or wait till another time. If you just can't get a strong test of the indicator muscle in the clear, you may want to turn to Chapter 10 for suggestions about how to find someone experienced in these procedures who can help out.

When you act as Subject for these procedures, it is important to remember that muscle testing is not a test of your strength or your health or your character. As you will see, it is perfectly normal for your muscles to become weak when something interferes with your body's energy, as we will explain in the next chapter. Don't feel compelled to use all your strength to fight against the Tester's pressure on your arm. If you notice yourself straining, clenching your teeth, or holding your breath, most likely you are trying too hard. Just relax, and allow yourself to go with the experience. You will be surprised at what you will learn about how your body works.

Four Simple Muscle Tests

Let's assume that you have gotten a strong test of the indicator muscle. Now you can go on to demonstrate muscle testing under various circumstances.

"Yes" and "No". First, the Subject should say "Yes" out loud. Test the muscle at the same time. It should remain strong on testing. Now have the Subject say "No," and test the muscle at the same time. The muscle should now test weak. This change in muscle strength will probably come as a surprise to you, if you are not already familiar with muscle testing. Once you get over the initial surprise of this simple demonstration, you will find that you can repeat this effect over and over.

Pinching and unpinching. Next try "pinching" and "unpinching" the muscle being tested. Begin by broadly and gently pinching the muscle along the side of the upper arm, one or two inches below the top of the shoulder, as shown in Illustration 4A. After this pinching procedure the muscle should test weak. Now unpinch the muscle by moving the fingers apart rather than squeezing them together; press against the muscle firmly (see Illustration 4B). Retest; the muscle should now test strong. Unpinching the muscle requires a delicate touch. If you don't find that it restrengthens the muscle, have the Subject simply move the arm around for a few seconds, and this will strengthen the muscle once again. This is the most difficult of the tests, so if it doesn't work well for you, just skip this one.

True and false name. For the next simple demonstration of muscle testing, have the Subject say, "My name is . . .," giving his or her correct name. Because the Subject is making an accurate statement, the arm muscle should test strong. Now have the Subject say, "My name is . . .," giving a false name. The arm muscle should now test weak. If you have never done muscle testing before, this will be a very impressive demonstration of the way that muscle testing works.[2]

Hand over navel. Now for a final demonstration of muscle testing, have the person place the palm of one hand over the navel while the muscle is being tested. If the arm is strong, then the energy is adequately balanced. This is actually the most sensitive test of all. After you have more experience, this test alone will probably suffice.

---

[2] It may appear from these procedures that muscle testing can be used as a "lie detector." Like a lie detector, muscle testing can be used to detect stress; however, it can give misleading results when used by inexperienced persons. Accurate use of muscle testing as a stress detector requires more advanced techniques, beyond the scope of this book.

These four simple procedures help to assure that the arm muscle is indicating properly. When you obtain the results as described, you are ready to go on to do allergy testing.

Special Energy Balancing Procedure

If you don't get the proper muscle responses on the above four tests, perform the following Special Energy Balancing procedure. You will be tapping a series of spots, in the same manner we have already described for the Energy Balancing Procedure above. Refer to the illustrations indicated for help in locating these spots on the body. In describing reflex point locations, "inner edge" of toes and fingers (with palms down) means towards the middle, or body midline.

1.a.Tap spots **2R & 2L** (right and left cheekbone, just below the center of eye); **3R & 3L** (outer edge of right and left second toe, just below the nail); **4R & 4L** (on the right and left side, at level halfway between crease of elbow and armpit); **5R & 5L** (inner edge of right and left big toe, just below the nail). All these spots are shown in Illustrations 5A, B, and C.

b. Next, touch lightly and continuously for about 30 seconds each of the following: Area 6 (mid-lower back at belt level) simultaneously with spots **7R & 7L** (inside edge of right and left index finger at base of nail; see Illustrations 6A and 6B); and then area 8 (along center of breastbone) simultaneously with spots **9R & 9L** (on the side of the thumb away from the fingers, at the base of the nail; see Illustrations 7A and 7B).

c. Next, touch lightly and hold for about 30 seconds, as above, spot **10** (top of skull, at end of middle finger when palm is placed on bridge of nose). The location of this spot is shown in Illustrations 8A, B, and C.

2.To check the results of this procedure, do the following Special Muscle Test:

Using either of Subject's arms, do the regular muscle test as above. Then, testing the Subject's same arm, Tester uses the other hand.

For example, if for the regular muscle test the Subject's left arm is used for testing, then ordinarily the Tester's right hand is used to press the Subject's arm. Now the Tester switches hands and tests the Subject's left arm with Tester's left hand. It takes longer to describe it than to do it! If the same arm tests strong using either hand, then go on to step 4. If the same arm tests weak using one hand and strong with the other hand, then also do the next Special Balancing Procedure.

3. Touch lightly and hold for about 30 seconds spots **11L** & **12L** simultaneously, and then **11R** & **12R** simultaneously (see Illustrations 9A and 9B); *or* **13L** & **14L** simultaneously, and then **13R** & **14R** simultaneously (see Illustrations 10A and 10B). Spots 11 (inside edge of foot, 1/3 distance between ball of foot and back of heel) and 12 (inside upper leg, 1/4 distance between knee and crotch) are very slightly better but less convenient than spots 13 (just above crook of elbow, outside edge of arm) and 14 (base of thumb, outside edge, center of fleshy part).

The regular Energy Balancing Procedure plus this Special Procedure will be adequate 99.9% of the time.

4. After performing this Special Energy Balancing Procedure (if necessary), go back and repeat the Four Simple Muscle Tests again. All the responses should now be as described.

Rechecking Balancing and Avoiding Fatigue

Whenever you do any muscle testing, remember that the indicator muscle must be properly balanced. From time to time during any testing session, be sure to go back and perform at least one of the Four Simple Muscle Tests, in order to make sure that the indicator muscle is still strong and properly balanced. Also, don't attempt to do too much in any one testing session because the muscle can become fatigued. Fifteen or 20 minutes is usually a realistic length for a session. In your enthusiasm when you begin muscle testing, you may overdo it. Excessive muscle testing may cause the arm to be a little sore for a couple of days, but has not otherwise been shown harmful. If you alternate testing between the right and the left arm from time to time, you will also help to avoid fatigue.

Muscle Testing in Lying Position

Up to this point we have described muscle testing in a standing position, but in actual practice when you are using muscle testing to deal with allergies, it is often much more convenient for the Subject to be lying down. The procedure for the lying position is essentially the same as for standing, except that the Subject in the lying position holds the arm straight up from the body at an angle of about 30 to 60 degrees, rather than out to the side (see Illustration 11). (Larger angles are better for people with weak muscles, and smaller angles for people whose muscles are strong.) The Tester presses straight down on the extended arm. It will probably feel a little different than in the standing position, so be sure to experiment with this position until you are familiar with how it feels.

Emotional Reactions Can Influence Muscle Testing

Sometimes when you think you're doing everything right, you may still get the "wrong" results, not because you're not properly energy balanced, but because there is an emotional involvement between the Subject and the Tester, or because either the Subject or the Tester has an unconscious emotional investment in making the test come out "wrong" (or "right," depending on your point of view). For this reason you may find it difficult to do muscle testing on close family members, your partner, your boss, or anyone with whom you have a strong emotional connection. You may find it better to work with a more neutral partner—a neighbor or friend or more distant relative.

ALLERGY TESTING

Once you are confident that you know how to do muscle testing, you can go on to test for allergies. Later on, in Appendix D, we will describe in detail how to collect samples of various substances for testing. But for now, simply select a food or other substance to which you think you might be allergic. If you think you might be allergic to wheat, you can use a slice of bread—but remember that bread contains more than just wheat, and later when you "fine tune" your allergy testing you will learn to sort out all the different ingredients. Or, if you want to test yourself for milk allergy, put a little milk in a closed container (to avoid spilling). If you suspect you are allergic to cats, get someone to collect some cat hair and put it in a plastic bag or a small jar. When you test for allergies, it usually doesn't matter whether the substance being tested is sealed or open to the air. If you are allergic to it, the test will usually work either way. However, using a closed container will help to prevent allergic reactions to a substance to which a person is very sensitive.

The allergy testing is done with two people, the Tester and the Subject. The Subject may be standing, sitting, or lying down, but the lying position is the most convenient. Be sure that the indicator muscle in the arm is strong to begin with, and that it is energy balanced if it does not test strong in the clear.

Allergy Test Spots. To test for allergies, you will use what we call the Allergy Test Spots, which are located just in front of the ear (see Illustrations 12A and 12B). You need to touch only one of these spots, either on the right or the left, and either the Tester or the Subject can touch the spot. We will describe one possible arrangement for doing this testing; but remember that either the Tester or the Subject can touch the spot. Touch the Test Spot only while muscle testing is actually being performed, so as not to fatigue the reflex. You only need to touch it lightly; there's no need to exert pressure.

First you want to test the strength of the indicator muscle while touching the Allergy Test Spot in the clear—that is, before the subject is exposed to a possible allergic substance. While the Allergy Test Spot is being touched, the Tester tests the Subject's arm to make sure that the muscle is indicating properly. The muscle should test strong.

A very few people will test weak, simply from touching the Allergy Test Spot. If this should happen to you, use the following procedure to strengthen the muscle.

1. Gently tap BOTH Allergy Test Spots (spots **15R** & **15L**, in front of the ear; see Illustrations 12A and 12B), on the right and the left side (either one at a time or simultaneously). These spots should be tapped for about 30 seconds, about 90 times.

2. Tap the Muscle Strengthening Spots (spots **16R** & **16L**), just above the crook of the elbow, on both the right and left upper arm, in the same manner as described above. (See Illustration 13).

If you follow these procedures and the indicator muscle still tests weak when the Subject touches the Allergy Test Spot, discontinue testing for the time being. Wait until another day, or repeat the testing with another person acting as Tester. An emotional interchange may be interfering with the testing procedure. Once again, if you can't solve the problem, see Chapter 10 for information about how to find help.

Testing with the test substance. Once the indicator muscle tests strong, you can go on to expose the Subject to the test substance. Place the substance (in a container, or by itself) on the Subject's abdomen just below the navel. This location we call the Substance Placement Area, or SPA (area **17**); we will be using it throughout these allergy and tolerance procedures for placing test substances (see Illustration 14A). If the Subject is lying down, the substance can of course just be placed on the abdomen, as shown in Illustration 14B. If the Subject is sitting or standing, either person can hold it in position, or it can be tucked under the belt or waistband.

Now have the Subject touch the Allergy Test Spot, and with the test substance in position on the Substance Placement Area test the Subject's arm again. If the muscle now tests weak, the Subject *is allergic* to the substance being tested. If the muscle tests strong, the Subject is *not allergic* to the test substance.[3] Until you are used to muscle testing, you may want to repeat this procedure a couple of times, just to make sure that your observations are accurate. Once you are sure that you are getting

---

[3] Note that even though a person may not be allergic to a substance, their tolerance for that substance may be quite small. See Chapter 4 for a discussion of tolerance and how to (sometimes) increase it.

consistent results with one test substance, go on to try another. When you have identified a substance to which the Subject is allergic, you will be ready to go on the Allergy Tap balancing method described in Chapter 3. However, before using this method you must be sure it will work for this substance and this Subject. A brief test for this purpose is described in the next chapter.

For those of you who are impatient and would like to learn the entire set of allergy correction procedures without the explanations of how they work, turn to Appendix A. Here you will find all the procedures in this book described completely. While we strongly recommend that you read the appropriate chapters before trying out the techniques, if you carefully follow the instructions in Appendix A you will get the right results.

How You Can Use This Book with Others

Almost everyone has allergies, some worse than others. You can use this book to help your family, your friends, and your fellow workers correct the allergies that are causing them discomfort and distress. When people get rid of their allergies, they may experience many benefits, such as:

—getting rid of uncomfortable symptoms
—having more energy
—living a less restricted lifestyle
—being able to get along better with others
—having more comfortable pregnancies and healthier babies

For many people, allergies have such a great influence that getting rid of their allergies enables them to live happier, more satisfying lives.

Learning to use the energy techniques described in this book can help to bring your family closer together. In an age when family members are being pulled in many different directions by conflicting interests and needs, it is valuable to take some time for a cooperative, loving, and healing exchange of energy.

It's not just your family members who can benefit from getting rid of their allergies. The same goes for the people in your workplace. Get your fellow workers involved. Practice these simple procedures with them. You may find they are happier, healthier, and more energetic, and you may find that your workplace is more harmonious as a result.

Even your pets will be healthier if you use the procedures described in this book! Through a method known as *surrogate testing*, discussed in Chapter 5, you can test infants, young children, debilitated people, even animals, and eliminate most, if not all, of their allergy problems.

2

Allergy And Your Body's Energy

The Changing Definition of Allergy

Allergy was known as far back as the ancient Egyptians, who recognized that stinging insect bites could be deadly for people who were sensitive to them. Over time allergy came to be defined as an *acquired abnormal reaction to a substance which is harmless for most people, but which causes uncomfortable or even dangerous symptoms for the allergic person.*

Eventually the medical concept of allergy became more restricted. According to the orthodox medical view, allergy develops as a result of repeated or excessive exposure to a specific substance, or *antigen*. In response to this substance, the body's immune system produces proteins known as *antibodies* which specifically match the antigen in question. When the body is exposed to a certain antigen, it produces huge quantities of the corresponding antibody, which lock onto the antigen molecules, triggering chemical reactions in the body's cells to disable or destroy the antigen. It is these chemical reactions that are responsible for allergic symptoms such as swelling, pain, itching, redness, or mucus production.

The antigen-antibody allergy model was introduced into medicine in the 1920s, based largely on research on inhaled allergic substances such as pollens or molds, which often *do* involve antibody reactions in the blood. However, antigen-antibody reactions are only a very small part of the whole range of allergic reactions. In many cases of allergy, especially those involving foods and chemicals, an antigen-antibody reaction does not necessarily occur. Such environmental sensitivities became the subject of a new field known as *clinical ecology.* Clinical ecologists now recognize that certain environmental substances, sometimes in very small quantities, can trigger a variety of reactions, many of which were not previously recognized as allergic, such as emotional problems, hyperkinetic behavior in children, and psychological and physical problems. Because conventional medicine has clung to the antigen-antibody model of allergy, it has been unable to deal with many forms of allergies, while at the same time it refuses to recognize that alternative approaches can be effective in these other cases.[4]

Energy Concept of Allergy

Although clinical ecology has introduced some valuable tools for identifying and treating allergy, its testing methods may still miss some allergic reactions, and its theory does not adequately explain why the body becomes allergic in the first place.

In my work I use a new definition of allergy: *a disturbance of the normal flow and balance of energy within the body when it is exposed to a given substance.*

In order to understand how the allergic body is different from the non-allergic one, we must look at the body in terms of the energy that flows through it.

In our culture we do not have a precise vocabulary for talking about this vital energy that suffuses all living things. The Chinese call it *Chi*, the Japanese *Ki*, the Hindus *prana*. In the West it has sometimes been called the "life force" or "vital force."

The ancient Chinese system of acupuncture makes practical use of this concept of energy. The Chi energy is believed to flow along specific pathways in the body known as meridians. Sickness is viewed as a derangement

---

4 The concepts in this chapter are discussed in greater detail in my book *Energy, Allergy, and Your Health.*

of the energy flow along these meridians. When acupuncture needles are inserted at specific points along the meridians, they affect, or balance, the energy flow, influencing mental and physical health. Recent scientific research in the West, using sensitive electronic instruments or radioactive tracer isotopes, has shown that these meridians have a real, physical existence.

Our body's energy is not limited just to the energy that flows through the meridians. Every cell in the body is a bundle of energy. As modern physics teaches, energy is the fundamental principle that underlies everything that happens in our bodies, including biochemical changes that occur within the cells. In one sense, any kind of disease or malfunction can be seen as an energy disturbance. When we say allergy is an energy disturbance, we mean that when there is allergy the flow of energy is blocked, disturbed, or unbalanced, and that as a result the biochemical processes do not proceed as they should.

It is the flow of energy in the body that regulates and controls all bodily processes, including the body's utilization of nutritional substances, the functioning of the immune system, and other bodily systems. In this view, when the immune system produces antibodies to a specific antigen, it is because there is already a disturbance in the body's energy and in the metabolic and chemical processes that it regulates. Antibody formation is simply a later stage of defense which the body mounts to cope with severe disturbances of metabolic function.[5]

This concept of allergy as energy disturbance was essential to the development of the techniques in this book. However, you do not need to "believe in" this energy concept in order for these Energy Balancing methods to work for you.

---

[5] In fact, I think the antigen-antibody reaction is "simply" a result of the overload of the tissues.

Why Muscle Testing Works to Reveal Allergies

Other methods of allergy testing. Traditional methods of testing for allergy have never been very reliable. Medical allergists generally depend on *skin testing*, in which a very small amount of the suspect substance is introduced into the person's skin through a scratch or an injection. If there is a reaction at the test site the person is considered allergic to that substance. Skin testing is not very helpful in identifying allergies to foods[6] and some other kinds of substances; after all, it is not normal to inject foods under the skin, and it is not surprising that there would be a reaction. In *sublingual testing*, used especially by clinical ecologists, a tiny amount of an extract of a test substance is placed under the person's tongue. If the test is positive, symptoms may appear very rapidly, including dramatic mental and behavioral reactions. *Cytotoxic testing* is a form of blood testing that has recently come into use by many nutritionally-oriented health professionals. In this method, an extract of the substance is mixed with a sample of the person's blood, which is then observed under a microscope for changes in the white cells. Since foods and other allergic substances do not normally get into the blood in this manner, it is no surprise that cytotoxic testing is not very reliable either.[7]

One simple method for determining food allergies is *pulse testing*. It has been observed that if you eat something to which you are allergic, your pulse rate will speed up. Another way to test for food allergies is through *dietary testing*, beginning either with a fast or with the elimination of suspect foods, then reintroducing foods, one at a time, to see if there is any reaction.

---

[6] This was shown definitively by research done in the 1930s.

[7] About 75% "reproducibility" is claimed for cytotoxic testing. My experience has indicated that the person must have been very recently exposed to a substance in order for it to "show up" as an allergic problem with cytotoxic testing. It is not clear how reliable the method is after prolonged exposure to allergens.

While all these methods of allergy testing have their uses, they may fail to identify many allergies.

Muscle testing. In Chapter 1, you observed for yourself how muscle testing can reveal allergies to specific substances. Muscle testing works by tapping into the body's energy system, enabling you to identify allergic substances that are interfering with the body's energy flow. Unlike the traditional allergy testing methods, muscle testing does not require that you observe an actual allergic response. If a substance is able to weaken the muscle being tested, you can deduce that the energy is being disturbed, and that the person is allergic to that substance. Thus, muscle testing is a highly sensitive method which is able to identify allergies whose effects are not directly observable.

How is muscle testing able to detect the body's sensitivity to a given substance? All objects in our environment are made up of a web of energy within their cells or molecules. This energy radiates out from each object in a field that interacts with the energy fields of other objects (just like magnets), including our own bodies. Thus any substance to which we are exposed is giving off an energy field that is able to interact with our own energy field. We already know that our bodies are capable of sensing many forms of energy—for example, the color of light or the pitch of a sound. It seems that our bodies are also able to recognize other energies that we have not yet been able to precisely measure and define.

Energy Techniques for Correcting Allergies

If you already know you have allergy problems, you are most likely familiar with some of the traditional methods for treating allergies. The most obvious approach is to avoid contact with the allergic substance—whether it is a food, an inhaled pollen or mold, an environmental chemical, or any other material. However, it's not always possible to avoid exposure to the substances to which we are sensitive. During pollen season, an allergic person might have to live in a sealed room, breathing only filtered air. People who are particularly sensitive to cigarette smoke or smog may also find it hard to avoid these materials in their everyday activities. For people with multiple allergies, the problem is particularly acute. Some people have such a broad and dramatic range of food allergies that there are very few foods they can eat, which makes it difficult for them to obtain proper nutrition from their diet.

Gloria was such a person. Not only was she extremely sensitive to environmental chemicals and many pollens, but also to all grains, beans and peas, red meats, poultry, seafoods, dairy products, onions and garlic, most fruits, potatoes, tomatoes, and some other foods. She obviously had to avoid all processed foods, and could eat little but certain fresh vegetables and eggs. Although such a diet can be nutritious, the more any diet is restricted the more difficult it is to meet all metabolic requirements. However, by strictly avoiding these foods until her allergies could be corrected through energy methods, by taking nutritional supplements, and by changing her lifestyle, she was able to overcome these restrictions and now eats a "normal" diet.

Because it is so difficult to avoid exposure to some allergic substances, many people receive "desensitization shots" from a medical allergist. These consist of a series of injections of small amounts of an extract of the allergic substance. After receiving these shots over a period of time, the person no longer *seems* to react to the allergic substance. However, I believe that desensitization shots don't really eliminate allergies, but rather that they exhaust the immune system, reducing the body's ability to react to materials that are actually toxic. I have found through muscle testing that people who have undergone desensitization shots may not show any overt reaction to a "formerly" allergic substance, but that the substance will still weaken their energy; and so the allergy, by our definition, is still present. Moreover, in my work with clients I have found that the materials used for desensitization shots are among the most toxic substances I have tested. This makes sense, considering that they are extracts of substances to which the person is allergic, even in normal concentrations. It is no wonder that repeated injections of these extracts wear down the immune system!

Many people with allergies also resort to a wide range of over-the-counter or prescription medications. These do nothing to resolve the underlying allergic problem, and often prolong the symptoms and/or depress immune system functioning. It's a high price to pay for symptom relief if you must be drowsy all the time, or suffer the dangerous side effects of cortisone-like drugs.

The techniques described in this book represent a revolutionary new approach to treating allergies. Instead of costly, uncomfortable desensitization shots, or the sometimes impossible task of avoiding allergic substances, or dosing yourself with harmful drugs, you can now rebalance and retune your body's energy to eliminate your allergies. After this energy balancing process has been performed, people report that they no longer have the allergic problems they had in the past. Even though the technique works only with the body's energy, the symptoms it relieves may include clearly-observed physical and psychological problems. Of course, it may take some time for the tissues to heal after the underlying allergy has been corrected; and, as we will discuss below, there may still be problems with "overloading" the system. Moreover, recovery from allergic problems is always most complete if energy balancing is accompanied by a sound program of diet and supplements, as described in my book *Energy, Allergy, and Your Health.*

The energy balancing technique consists of stimulating certain energy reflex points while being exposed to the substance to which you are allergic. The process generally takes only a few minutes for each substance. This energy balancing technique works for all kinds of allergies—to foods, pollens, molds, perfumes, chemicals, pollutants, natural gas, and so on.

For example, Sheila, a young art student, came to me with multiple sensitivities to the solvents, chemicals, resins, and other materials encountered at her art school. When she entered the building, she would get a headache, making it very difficult for her to work. After we did the energy balancing procedures, she was able to go to school without getting headaches.

Another of my clients, Barbara, was scheduled to attend a program at an alcoholic halfway house. Although she was highly motivated to recover from her alcoholism problem, she found that at the meetings most people smoked cigarettes very heavily, and whenever she breathed in the cigarette smoke she would get a terrible, persistent pain in her chest. Before she went to her next meeting we did the energy balancing technique while she was being exposed to tobacco smoke. She was able to go to her program, and had no reaction to the cigarette smoke there. Note, however, that eliminating the allergy does not make the smoke any less toxic.

Some people are so severely allergic that they can only function properly in special environments. When we identify the things to which they are allergic and do the energy balancing process, they are able to live in less restricted environments without adverse reactions. This can be especially important for people who are allergic to substances that they encounter regularly in their workplace.

In my practice, I have observed that serious tissue pathology may improve after using these energy balancing techniques. Many symptoms that you might not think were allergic in nature—such as uterine fibroids, cancer, arthritis, or so-called autoimmune diseases—have cleared up completely after the use of these techniques (accompanied by a nutritional program).

Keep in mind that the simplified methods presented in this book will work only about 90% of the time. More extreme allergies are generally the ones *not* corrected by these methods. See Chapter 10 for information about finding a professional trained in an even more effective approach called Symbiotic Energy Transformation™ (SET).

The SET energy balancing techniques that I have been using in my practice are quite complex, and require a thorough knowledge of the reflex points involved, as well as the ability to determine which points to use. However, now with the simpler version described in this book, which I call the Allergy Tap, the vast majority of readers will be able to correct their allergies on their own, working with a friend.

Once you have learned how to do muscle testing, as described in Chapter 1, next determine whether the Allergy Tap method will work for you.

Finding Out Whether the Allergy Tap Will Work for You

To determine whether you are in the 90 percent who can be helped by the Allergy Tap method, follow the procedure described below. In actual practice, once you have learned the Allergy Test procedure described in Chapter 1, when you identify a substance to which the Subject is allergic you should immediately follow the Allergy Test procedure with the Allergy Tap Test below, to determine whether the Allergy Tap procedure will work for that substance. With a given person the Allergy Tap might work for one substance but not for another. Now here is the Allergy Tap Test.

Allergy Tap Test

1. It will be most convenient for the Subject to be lying down, as for allergy testing as described in Chapter 1. Make sure that the indicator muscle in the Subject's arm is strong; if necessary, balance the muscle as described under Muscle Testing in Chapter 1.

2. First test the Subject in the clear, as follows. Lightly touch the Allergy Tap Underarm Test Spots in the armpits, as shown in Illustrations 15A and 15B. Make sure that both Underarm Test Spots are touched—one by the Tester and one by the Subject. Illustrations 15A and 15B show the Tester Touching one spot; the Subject can touch the other. These spots should be touched only during the actual muscle testing, using only light pressure. If the indicator muscle tests strong (without exposure to the test substance), continue on with step 3. If the indicator muscle is weak, strengthen it with the following procedure.

   a. Lightly touch spots **19R** and **19L** simultaneously for 30 seconds. These spots are on the center of the inside of the right and left wrist, as shown in Illustration 16.

   b. Retest the indicator muscle in the arm. The muscle should now be strong. If not, wait until another time, or seek help as described in Chapter 10.

3. Now test the Subject, while he or she is being exposed to the test substance. As in the Allergy Test method described in Chapter 1, place the test substance over the Substance Placement Area (spot **17**), on the Subject's abdomen just below the navel. The Tester tests the Subject's arm muscle while the Underarm Test Spots (spots **18L** & **18R**) are being touched, as shown in Illustrations 15A and 15B. If the muscle tests *weak* on exposure, the Allergy Tap *will work* for this person and this substance. If the muscle tests *strong*, the Allergy Tap will *not work* to eliminate the Subject's allergy to the test substance, and the longer SET method will need to be performed by a qualified professional. (Again, Chapter 10 will provide suggestions about how to find an appropriate professional.)

The Simpler the Substance, the Better the Results

If the Allergy Tap Test indicates that the Allergy Tap will *not* work for the test substance, it may be that too many different materials are combined in the test item.   If the Subject tests allergic to wheat bread but testing shows that the Allergy Tap won't work for wheat bread as a whole, test separately for the different ingredients—wheat berries, yeast, etc.—both to identify the specific substance(s) to which the Subject is allergic, and to determine whether the Allergy Tap will work for that substance.   The narrower the range of substances being tested, the greater is the chance the Allergy Tap will work to correct an allergy to it.   If the Allergy Tap Test indicates that the Allergy Tap won't work, don't give up on the whole process.   It does not necessarily mean that the Allergy Tap won't work at all for this person.   Try simpler substances, or other kinds of substances, and see if the Allergy Tap will work for them.

3

How To Cure Your Allergies In Minutes

Once you have identified a substance to which you are allergic, and for which the Allergy Tap method will work, you are ready to use this Allergy Tap for solving most of your allergy problems.

If you are still unsure about what kinds of substances to collect and test for allergy, see Appendix D, which explains in detail how to collect samples and how to prepare them for testing and energy balancing.

What might you expect as a result of using the Allergy Tap to correct your allergies? For some people the results are truly spectacular. About a year ago I worked with a young woman who was just entering the eleventh grade in high school. All her life Joan had suffered from severe asthma and other serious allergic problems. Every year she would miss about 20 days of school because of illness, and her asthma prevented her from engaging in sports and other vigorous activities. Over the years her parents had spent thousands upon thousands of dollars on allergy testing, desensitization shots, and other medical care. About a year ago, I spent a total of two or three hours with Joan, doing some of the simple Allergy Tap procedures. When I saw her again recently, her entire life had changed. She had stopped going to the medical allergist, was no longer taking allergy shots, and had become physically active to the point that she had made the girls' volleyball team at school. Joan was bubbling over with enthusiasm for the energy methods we had used. She had been subjected to traditional allergy approaches all her life without relief, and now she was able to live a normal life.

Your results may not be as spectacular as Joan's, but hopefully you will be able to see some real, demonstrable effects from using the Allergy Tap method to correct your own allergic problems. Now, here are the step-by-step instructions for the Allergy Tap. Remember that for future reference the complete instructions for muscle testing, allergy testing and balancing, and tolerance testing and balancing are contained in Appendix A. All the reflex points are detailed in the easy-to-use reference chart in Appendix C.

THE ALLERGY TAP PROCEDURE

In Chapter 1 you learned how to use muscle testing to find a substance to which you are allergic, and in Chapter 2 you learned the test to determine whether the Allergy Tap method would work for a given substance and a given Subject. Now, once you have identified a substance to which you or another Subject is allergic, and for which the Allergy Tap will work, you can go on to perform the Allergy Tap to eliminate the allergy to that substance.

The Subject may be sitting, standing, or lying down for this procedure, but the lying position is generally easier. Since you will need to touch some spots on the feet, the Subject's shoes, and preferably socks,[8] should be removed.

---

[8] The only reason to remove the socks is to be able to see the precise location of the reflex points. Once you are sure you know exactly where the points are located, removal of the socks is unnecessary.

Exposure to Test Substance

Using a sample of the substance to which the Subject has been shown to be allergic, expose the Subject to the test substance. Unlike the allergy testing procedure, exposure to the substance might now be *enhanced*. Instead of simply placing it in a closed container on the Substance Placement Area below the navel, the Subject could now be exposed to the substance in a manner similar to that encountered in everyday experience. For example, if the substance is a food, a little could be placed in the mouth. If it is a perfume or some other inhaled substance, it could be gently sniffed. If it is a chemical or a cosmetic, it could be touched or applied to the skin. BE CAREFUL, however, if the Subject is known or suspected to be extremely allergic to the test substance. In this case it is preferable to keep it in a closed container while the Allergy Tap procedure is being done. Once the Subject's sensitivity to the substance has been reduced through this procedure, you can repeat the Allergy Tap, if necessary, with enhanced exposure to the substance, though this is rarely necessary. If you are not sure about a substance, keep it in a closed container. As the Allergy Tap usually works for less severe allergies, it is unlikely that the procedure will work if the person is highly sensitive to a substance.

Tapping Spots

Now, while the Subject is being exposed to the substance as we have described above, eight sets of Tapping Spots are lightly tapped with the fingertips. Either the Subject or the Tester can tap the spots, and in any order. Note that both people can tap points simultaneously, saving time. We will describe one possible arrangement in detail, but you can vary it as you wish, as long as all spots are tapped on both the right and the left sides. Tap each set of Tapping Spots, right and left, for 30 seconds, about 35 times. You may tap both right and left simultaneously. Spots 20, 21, 22, and 23 (right and left) may be tapped simultaneously in any combination and any order, as may Spots 2, 3, 4, and 5 (right and left). You may recognize Spots 2—5 as the spots previously used for energy balancing in Chapter 1. Now, we will go over one possible version of the tapping procedure in detail, for each set of spots.

1. Gently tap Spots **20R** and **20L,** which are located at the right and left side of the bridge of the nose, at the inner corner of the eye. Be careful not to injure the eye. Next tap Spots **21R** and **21L,** on the outer edge of the right and left little toe, just below the nail. These spots are shown in Illustrations 17A and 17B.

2. Tap Spots **22R** and **22L,** right and left sides of the breastbone at the junction of the collarbone and the first rib. Next tap Spots **23R** and **23L,** in the center of the ball of the foot on each foot. These spots are shown in Illustrations 17A and 17C.

3. Tap Spots **2R** and **2L,** on the cheekbones just below the center of the right and the left eye, again being careful not to injure the eye. Next tap Spots **3R** and **3L,** on the outer edge of the right and left second toe, just below the nail. These spots are shown in Illustrations 5A and 5B.

4. Finally, tap Spots **4R** and **4L,** on the right and left sides of the body, at a level halfway between the crease of the elbow when the arm is bent, and the armpit. The Subject can tap both these points simultaneously by crossing the arms and tapping the opposite sides, as shown in Illustration 5C. Meanwhile, tap Spots **5R** and **5L,** on the inner edge of the right and left big toe, just below the nail, shown in Illustration 5B.

That's all there is to it. You have now completed the Allergy Tap procedure for this substance, and you may go on to retest for allergy to verify that the Subject now tests strong.

Retesting for Allergy

Go back to the Allergy Test procedure described in Chapter 1, using the same substance for which you just did the Allergy Tap. If the Subject's arm now tests strong when exposed to the test substance, the allergy has been eliminated. If the Subject's exposure to the substance has been limited up to this point—for example, if it has been enclosed in a container—you may now want to repeat the Allergy Test with a stronger exposure to the substance;[9] if on testing the Subject still shows sensitivity to the substance, you should repeat the Allergy Tap with more direct exposure, although this is rarely needed.   In any case it is a good idea to wait a few days before repeating the procedure because often the Subject continues to improve for some time after the method has been done.

If the Subject tests weak when exposed to the substance, you will need to figure out what went wrong.   If you suspect that you may not have tapped the Tapping Spots adequately, review the instructions and repeat the procedure if necessary.   You may not have done the Allergy Tap Test correctly, as described in Chapter 2.   In either case, test the indicator muscle in the clear, without exposure to the test substance.   If it tests weak, rebalance the muscle and repeat the Allergy Tap Test.   If the test still indicates that the Allergy Tap will work, repeat the Allergy Tap procedure.

If in spite of all your efforts you still can't get the Allergy Tap to work correctly, follow the suggestions in Chapter 10 for finding help.

Don't Fix Too Much at One Time

Doing the Allergy Tap for allergy is so simple that you may be tempted to try to correct all of a person's allergies in one session.   However, it's better to go about correcting allergies slowly and gradually.   Many serious ailments, such as tumors or other tissue disorders, may be related to allergies, and when the allergies are corrected the diseased tissues begin to break down and be reabsorbed by the body.   If too many serious problems are resolving at the same time, the lymph system can become clogged up, resulting in pain and discomfort.   The person may have serious tissue pathology without even knowing it, but when it begins to clear up they feel the resulting discomfort. Especially if you are aware that the person has serious health problems, be very careful in doing allergy correction work, working with no more than one or two allergic substances in any one day.   Even so, remember that the more serious allergies usually require the SET technique.   Proper use of the Allergy Tap Test will help you avoid correcting too much at one time.   When the

---

[9]   But remember that the person's *tolerance* may still be low, so don't overdo it.

person has "had enough" the test will indicate no correction is to be done. Later, when the body is ready, the Allergy Tap Test will indicate the correction may now be completed. This is why repeating the Allergy Tap Test again later, for every substance originally not correctable, is a good idea. Over time, as the body gets healthier, allergies to most or perhaps all allergic substances might be correctable.

The Healing Process

After you have used the Allergy Tap to correct your allergies, your body will begin to go through what is known as a *healing process*. During this process you may experience uncomfortable symptoms, such as a reduction of energy, a need to sleep more, various aches and pains, digestive disturbances, or increased secretions.

Once you have removed the energy blocks that were responsible for your allergies, the tissues affected by the allergies begin to heal and to function better. As tissue function improves, toxic substances are released from the cells and tissues and are dumped into the system, making the body temporarily more toxic. This is partly what produces the symptoms of the healing reaction. Similarly, people who have used "recreational drugs" such as cocaine or marijuana sometime in the past may experience symptoms that mimic the effects of these drugs, as the drug residues stored in the tissues are released.

People whose systems are very toxic, or who have severe tissue damage, are likely to experience the strongest healing reactions. This is why you are urged to go slowly in your use of the Allergy Tap method, and not try to do too much at one time. As described above, proper use of the Allergy Tap Test will minimize any such effects.

When your allergy to a certain substance is eliminated, your body will no longer need to produce mucus to protect itself against that substance, and so you will begin to clear the mucus out of your body. As a result, you may even find that you cough a great deal. You may also have increased urination or unpleasant body odors. These symptoms do not mean that something is wrong, but rather that toxic materials are being released from the body's cells.

In the course of the healing process old symptoms may reappear. This doesn't mean that you are getting worse, but rather that your body is moving to a better state of health. If you know ahead of time that you may experience the return of these symptoms, you will be less likely to panic or believe you are getting sicker when they occur. If you take pain killers or antihistamines or other drugs to suppress these symptoms, you will simply prolong the healing process and cause the symptoms to last longer. Indeed, many people discover that these drugs simply have no effect on the symptoms. This is because there is nothing "wrong," so the drug has no place to act. This process can be quite puzzling until you understand what is happening. Be patient; it will pass soon.

The experience of one of my clients illustrates how difficult the healing process can be. Mona R. first came to my office hobbling along on a cane, moving with difficulty and in constant pain. Her arthritis had developed rapidly, and she looked at least ten years older than she was. In spite of the hopeless prognoses she had received from numerous health professionals, Mona was a fighter and was absolutely determined to overcome her affliction. Her high motivation helped her to follow closely the program we worked out for her. Now, only a year later, Mona is almost over her arthritis. She threw away her cane months ago, and her energy level is higher than she can remember in years. That is not to say that she is now "cured." There is much more healing and repair for the body to perform—a process that can take years more.

This transformation was not an easy process, however. In the course of healing her body, Mona experienced a very lengthy series of symptoms which most people, unaware of the healing process, would have interpreted as getting sicker. Mona had very low energy for a long time. At times she had severely swollen ankles, feet, and legs. For a while she hobbled even more than originally. She had an assortment of aches and pains which would drive most people to their physician for pain killers and tranquilizers. She had been warned, however, that she would reexperience many symptoms from years before, and soon she discovered that as these symptoms abated the affected body part became as good as new.

The "very low energy" mentioned above is the most common report from people who are going through a significant healing process. This seems to be because the body does not have available the resources to carry out the healing process and at the same time do all the usual daily "running around" that we usually do. The body simply cannot transport all the increased, and necessary, raw materials (nutrients), dispose of the greater amount of debris (from tearing down the inadequate tissue), and also maintain the usual level of other daily activity.

Symptoms are not a sign that something is awry, but rather that the body is at work correcting something which is wrong. If you fight the symptoms you are fighting the body.

As you use the Allergy Tap method, remember that such healing reactions may well occur. The less you try to do at any one time, the less severe these reactions will be. So, be prepared, don't panic, and go slow!

4

Allergy Versus Intolerance: It May Not Be Allergy

It May Not Be Allergy

Suppose that you have used the Allergy Tap to eliminate an allergy to a certain substance. Does that mean that you can now expose yourself to that substance without harm?

The answer is: not necessarily. We must strongly caution you that eliminating an allergy to a harmful substance, such as tobacco, does not make it OK to use that substance in the future. Part of the reason for this is that you will still have an *intolerance* to that substance. Indeed, no matter how pure, healthy, or nutritious a substance, we all will have a limited tolerance to it. Of course, that tolerance may be very high, but not necessarily so.

Because people have become so allergy-conscious nowadays, they often jump to the conclusion that *any* adverse reaction to foods or other environmental substances is due to allergy. However, there are many other reasons for such reactions, which may call for entirely different strategies in dealing with them.

Take the example of Alice, who brought her baby in to my office with a severe skin rash. The well-meaning pediatrician, assuming that the rash was due to a milk allergy, had placed the baby on soy formula. The rash got no better. In this youngster's case, the problem was not allergy at all, but severe digestive system deficiencies which prevented proper digestion of his food. Not only was the switch to soy formula depriving the baby of the beneficial substances in his mother's milk, but his problems continued until his symptoms were finally interpreted correctly.

Another example: After eating in a restaurant, Mark experienced chills and fever, nausea, and vomiting. Since he had a tendency to food allergies, he dismissed his symptoms as "just another allergic reaction," and did not seek treatment. In reality, Mark had a case of food poisoning from Salmonella. Had he sought help for this bacterial infection, he would have been spared much discomfort.

Many Forms of Intolerance

Both these cases are examples of intolerances. In connection with my nutritional consulting practice, I have identified more than a dozen reasons, other than allergy, why people may have adverse reactions to foods due to intolerances.[10] In a general sense, all these forms of intolerance are due to *overloading* the system with more of a substance than it can process. While I consider allergy to be a disturbance of the body's energy system, intolerances are primarily a disturbance of the body's metabolic/biochemical state. Even though intolerances operate on a biochemical level, I have found that many people can obtain help for some of their intolerances through a special set of energy techniques.

Benefits of Correcting Intolerances

Note that I say "many people" can obtain help. Whereas the Allergy Tap works to correct allergies 90 percent of the time, I have found that increases in tolerance can be obtained in only about 20 percent of all cases.

---

[10] For a complete discussion of these reasons for intolerance see my book *Energy, Allergy, and Your Health.*

I do not know any general rules about when the method will work. It may work for some people for certain substances and not for others, or it may be able to increase one person's tolerance for a given substance but provide no help for another person with the same substance. However, when the Tolerance Tap method described in this chapter does work for individuals, it can make a great deal of difference for them—sometimes the difference between being able to live in their own home or not. Our environments are filled with so many chemicals and other harmful materials, that if a highly sensitive person can increase his tolerance to such substances he may be able to live a much more comfortable and productive life.

Even if you are not able to *increase* your tolerance to a given substance, it is very useful simply to know what your *tolerance level* is. *Tolerance testing may be the single most important concept and technique you will learn in this book.*

If you knew what your tolerance level was for every substance with which you came into contact in your life, and if you never exceeded your tolerance level, you would be a much healthier, happier, more vital, and energetic person.

A good example of the importance of knowing your tolerance level is *water.* Most people need to drink about 50 to 70 ounces of water a day, but many sources of water, such as tap water, much well water, and even bottled water, contain many contaminants for which your tolerance may be very low. Using samples of whatever sources of water you regularly use, you can determine your tolerance levels. You may be surprised to discover that your tolerance for these water samples is so low that you cannot meet your daily need for water from these sources. If this is the case, then you must search for a water source, or a water purification system, that will provide a suitably adequate tolerance level. The best purification systems yield water that tests at a tolerance level of more than 200 ounces per day for most people. Anything less than 100 ounces or so is quite inadequate.

Just as you can test everything in your environment for allergy, so can you test your tolerance level. Test your tolerance not only for foods, but also for household items such as cleaning fluids, detergents, and cosmetics. Test the items in your medicine cabinet, including your medications. Appendix D will provide you with many more suggestions.

Knowing your tolerance levels can have far-reaching effects. For example, Marilyn always was concerned about her weight. She had difficulty sticking to any diet because she knew that afterwards her weight would return. At first, she had difficulty believing that the calories she ate weren't very important, but rather it was the quality of the food. After some practice and an agreement to try out the process for two weeks, she began to determine her tolerance level for *everything* she ate or drank, and vowed not to exceed those amounts. She did so, and was amazed to discover that losing weight was rather easy, did not require any real sacrifice, and did not cause her any discomfort. Now she never puts anything in her mouth she hasn't tested. She not only maintains her ideal weight, but she has more pep and energy than she ever thought she could have. Most importantly, she feels great!

In the instructions that follow, you will first learn how to test your tolerance level for whatever substance you select. You will then be shown a test to determine whether your tolerance for that substance can be increased through the Tolerance Tap method. If it cannot, you may retest with other substances, or perhaps with simpler forms of the substance previously tested—such as testing for wheat berries rather than whole wheat bread. Once you have identified a substance for which your tolerance can be increased, you can then use the Tolerance Tap; you will generally obtain a twofold to sixfold increase in your tolerance for that substance.

As a general rule, whenever you complete the Energy Balancing Procedure for correcting an allergy, immediately go on to test your tolerance level for the same substance. By keeping exposure below the tolerance level (and by increasing your tolerance level where possible), you will be able to avoid problems with the substance in question.

TOLERANCE TESTING AND TOLERANCE ENERGY BALANCING

Testing Your Tolerance Level

Just as you used muscle testing to determine whether you were allergic to specific substances, you can also use muscle testing to determine your tolerance level for a given substance, and in some cases you can increase your tolerance using an energy technique.

Test samples. When you used muscle testing to test for allergy, it didn't matter how much of the test substance was used. When you test for tolerance, the amount of the substance is a critical factor. In testing your tolerance for foods, it's good to begin with an average serving size. For example, if you are testing the Subject's tolerance for eggs, you might begin by exposing the Subject to one egg. If you are testing your tolerance to wheat, you could start with a tablespoon of wheat flour or wheat berries. For many substances it will help to use a small glass dish or other container, so that you can readily vary the amount being tested.

To test tolerance levels for inhaled substances, simply vary the amount of the substance you inhale. Begin with a very quick sniff, and if that tests OK, then cautiously increase up to a deep inhalation, if tolerated. **Be careful,** however; some substances are not safe to inhale except in the very smallest sniffs. For detailed instructions about testing inhalants, see the instructions in Appendix D. To repeat the warning given above, use closed containers first, and then very gradually increase exposure whenever any suspect item, or possibly toxic item, is being tested.

First make sure that the indicator muscle tests strong, and if necessary do energy balancing as described in Chapter 1. As with allergy testing, the Subject may be sitting, standing, or lying down, but if you are going to use a container to hold the test substance it will obviously be more convenient for the Subject to lie down (see Illustration 18). As with the allergy work, shoes and socks should be removed to afford access to the reflex spots on the feet.

Tolerance Test Spots. Begin by lightly touching one of the Tolerance Test Spots (**24RL**), which are located at either side of the back of the neck, as shown in Illustrations 19A and 19B. You don't need to touch both spots simultaneously, but only one. To be sure you touch the Tolerance Test Spot, place your fingertips lightly on the soft spot just under the skull on one side of the back of the neck. There is no need to exert pressure. As when you did allergy testing, don't touch the Tolerance Test Spot continuously, but only while muscle testing is actually being performed. This is to prevent the reflex spot from becoming fatigued.

First touch the Tolerance Test Spot and test the strength of the indicator muscle in the clear (without exposure to the test substance). The arm should test strong.

In rare cases the arm will test weak simply from touching the Tolerance Test Spot. To strengthen the arm muscle, use the following procedure:

a.Tap for 30 seconds (about 35 times) the Tolerance Test Spot Strengthening Point (spot 25R) on the inside edge of the right little finger at the base of the nail, while simultaneously touching spot 10 on the top of the head, at the point reached by the middle finger when the palm is placed on the bridge of the nose. (See Illustrations 20A and 20B.)

b.Repeat for Subject's left little finger (spot 25L) and spot 10.

c.Retest to make sure the arm now tests strong. If it does not, discontinue testing for the time being. If this situation persists, follow the suggestions in Chapter 10 to find help.

Once you have obtained a strong muscle test while the Tolerance Test Spots are being touched, you can proceed to the actual tolerance testing.

Tolerance testing. Place the selected amount of the test substance, either in a container or by itself, on the Substance Placement Area (spot 17) on the abdomen just below the navel, as shown in Illustrations 14A and 14B. This is the testing position shown in Illustration 18. Touch one of the Tolerance Test Spots (24R or 24L) with the test substance in place on the abdomen, and test the Subject's arm. If the muscle tests *strong*, this means that the Subject's tolerance for this substance is *greater* than the sample amount. In this case, increase the sample size and repeat the muscle test until you find the amount just slightly less than is required to weaken the indicator muscle. This is the *tolerance level*.

If the arm tests *weak*, the Subject's tolerance for this substance is *less* than the sample amount. Reduce the amount of the test substance and repeat muscle testing until you find the level at which the arm tests strong. This is the *tolerance level*.

Use common sense to decide how much to increase or decrease the amount of the test substance. If the arm tests strong with one egg, you can try two eggs and then four. If you need to reduce the amount of egg, you may need

to break it and separate out part of it, say a half. Or it might be more convenient to boil the egg and cut it in halves, thirds, or fourths. Of course,
with an egg, it might also be important to test the white and yolk separately, as it is common for a person to be allergic to only part of the egg.

CAN THE TOLERANCE LEVEL BE INCREASED FOR THIS PERSON AND THIS SUBSTANCE?

Tolerance Tap Test Spots. Once you have determined the Subject's tolerance for a given substance, you next need to determine whether the
Tolerance Tap can be used to increase the Subject's tolerance for that
substance. Begin by making sure once again that the indicator muscle is
strong, and rebalance it if necessary. Then have the Subject lie down
and touch both Tolerance Tap Test Spots (spots **4R** and **4L**), on the
right and left side of the torso at a level halfway between the crook of
the elbow when the arm is bent, and the armpit, as shown in Illustrations 21A and 21B. (These spots should be familiar to you, since they
were previously used for energy balancing and for correcting allergies.)
One convenient arrangement is for the Subject to place one hand over
the Tolerance Tap Test Spot on the same side as the arm being used for
muscle testing, while the Tester places a hand on the Test Spot on the
side opposite the arm being tested. The Tester then tests the Subject's
free arm.

If this test in the clear (without exposure to any substance) is strong, then
go on to the Tolerance Tap Test below. If the muscle tests weak to begin
with, strengthen it first by doing the following:

Touch and hold for about 30 seconds spots **26L** and **27L** simultaneously,
followed likewise by spots **26R** and **27R** simultaneously. Spots 26R and
26L are located at the corner of the jaw; spots 27R and 27L are located
on the forehead, straight above the center of the eye and on the bottom
edge of the "frontal eminence"—the small ridge running across the forehead about an inch and a half above the eyebrows (see Illustrations 22A
and 22B). (Another set of Tolerance Tap Test Spots is located on the
inner edge of the right and the left big toe, just below the nail, Spots
5R and **5L**, as shown in Illustration 5B. However, these spots are not

quite as effective as those on the sides and should be used only if the spots on the sides for some reason cannot conveniently be used.)

Tolerance Tap Test. Now expose the Subject to *any* amount of the substance, placing it on the Substance Placement Area as described above. Here the amount is not critical. With the test substance in place, touch the Tolerance Tap Test Spots and test the indicator muscle as previously described. If the arm muscle tests *weak* while the Tolerance Tap Test Spots are being touched and the Subject is being exposed to the test substance, the Subject's tolerance for this substance *can be increased* by the Tolerance Tap. If it tests *strong*, the Tolerance Tap *will not work* to increase the Subject's tolerance for this substance.

Remember that tolerance increase can be obtained in only about 20 percent of all cases, even using the long method administered by a qualified professional. The Tolerance Tap will work about 96 percent as well as the long method when it does work.

Tolerance Tap Procedure

If you have determined that the Tolerance Tap will work for a given substance, use the following procedure to increase the Subject's tolerance to that substance.

Expose the Subject to *any amount* of the substance, as described above. The Subject then places one palm over the navel area, Tolerance Area A (area **28**), shown in Illustrations 23A and 23B. (The area around the navel contains reflex points representing all of the meridians in the body's energy system. This is why this area is so effective when the palm is placed over it.)

With the Subject's palm covering Tolerance Area A, and with the test substance on the Substance Placement Area on the abdomen just below the navel, tap Tapping Spots 20 through 23, right and left, as described below. These spots are all shown in Illustrations 17A, B, and C. Tapping is continued for 30 seconds, about 35 times, for each set of spots. Any combination of Spots 20-23 may be tapped individually or simultaneously. These are the same

Tapping Spots that you previously used in the allergy correction procedure in Chapter 3.

a.Gently tap spots **20R** & **20L**, on both the right and the left side of the nose, at the inner corner of the eye (see Illustration 17A). Be careful not to injure the eye.

b.Tap spots **21R** & **21L**, on the outer edge of the right and left little toes, just below the nail (see Illustration 17B).

c.Tap spots **22R** & **22L**, on both sides of the breastbone at the junction of the collarbone, the first rib, and the breastbone (see Illustration 17A).

d.Tap spots **23R** and **23L**, in the center of the ball of the foot, on the right and left sole (see Illustration 17C).

Next the Subject places the right hand over Tolerance Area B (area 29), as shown in Illustrations 24A and 24B. The hand is placed over the left rib cage, with the little finger along the bottom of the ribs and the fingers spread slightly. The left hand can also be used, but in that case be sure that the same area on the left side is covered. See the illustration to see why it is necessary to spread the fingers to make sure that all the important spots are being covered.

Now, with the Subject covering Tolerance Area B, and with *any amount* of the substance still on the Substance Placement Area, tap spots 2 through 5, right and left sides, as described below. These spots are shown in Illustrations 5A, B, and C. Again, each set of spots is tapped gently for 30 seconds, or about 35 times; any combination of Spots 2-5, right and left, may be tapped simultaneously.

e.Gently tap spots **2R** & **2L**, on the cheekbones just below the center of the right and left eye (see Illustration 5A); be careful not to injure the eye.

f.Tap spots **3R** & **3L**, on the outer edge of the right and left second toe, just below the nail (see Illustration 5B).

g.Tap spots **4R** & **4L**, on the right and left sides at a level halfway between the crook of the elbow, arm bent, and the armpit (see Illustration 5C).

h.Tap spots **5R** & **5L**, on the inner edge of the right and left big toe, just below the nail (see Illustration 5B).

This completes the Tolerance Tap procedure. Now you can go on to retest the Subject's tolerance, to see how much it has been increased.

Retesting Tolerance Level

Test the indicator muscle once again to make sure it is still strong, and rebalance it if necessary. This time use an amount of the test substance *just larger* than the previously determined tolerance level, and repeat the tolerance test as described above. If the indicator muscle now tests strong for this amount, keep increasing the sample amount until you determine the new tolerance level. Generally you can expect to increase tolerance by two to six times the original level through the use of this Tolerance Tap, in cases where it is effective.

5

Surrogate Testing
And Treatment

Does your newborn infant have allergies? How much milk, or wheat, can your young child tolerate? Do you have an elderly or sick person in your home who is too weak to respond properly to muscle testing? Would you like to know if your pet is receiving an adequate diet?

All these questions can be addressed through a technique known as surrogate testing. The procedure is very simple. The only difference between using a surrogate and the techniques we have learned so far, is that *three* individuals are involved instead of two. These three are:

The Tester—the person doing the testing
The Surrogate—the person whose arm is being tested
The Subject—the person (or animal) being tested through the Surrogate by the Tester.

In surrogate testing, the Subject (whether a child, an adult, or an animal), is touched or held by the Surrogate. If the Subject is an infant, for example, the mother may act as the Surrogate, holding the infant in her arms or even nursing it. If the Subject is an elderly person in bed, the Surrogate may hold the Subject's hand or place a hand on the Subject's shoulder. Instead of the Tester doing muscle testing on the Subject, it is the Surrogate whose arm is tested. The Surrogate's muscle testing reflects the condition of the Subject who is being touched.

Before beginning surrogate testing for allergies or intolerances, make sure that both the Tester and the Surrogate are energy balanced, as well as the Subject, as described in Chapter 1, or Appendix A, Section IA.

Place the test substance at the proper Substance Placement Area on the abdomen of *either* the Subject *or* the Surrogate. The Allergy or Tolerance Test Spot can be touched on *either* the Subject *or* the Surrogate, although it is slightly preferable to touch the Subject's Test Spot if possible.

To correct allergies or increase tolerance, follow the normal procedure, except that the Surrogate is once again used for muscle testing. You can do the correction procedures (tapping the Tapping Spots) on *either* the Subject *or* the Surrogate. It is somewhat preferable to use the Tapping Spots on the Subject if possible, but it is not essential.

When these procedures are followed properly, the Surrogate's own allergies or intolerances do not interfere with the testing and correction process. If the Subject and the Surrogate are properly energy balanced, and if the Subject is being held or touched by the Surrogate, the Surrogate's own allergies and intolerances simply do not enter into the situation. You may want to try some experiments to demonstrate this for yourself. Acting as Tester, test a friend (Subject #1) for allergies. Then test another friend (Subject #2) who does not have the same allergies. Have Subject #1 touch Subject #2, acting as #2's Surrogate, and you will observe that muscle testing on the Surrogate now demonstrates Subject #2's allergies, rather than the Surrogate's own allergies. Now reverse the roles and you will find that the opposite is true also.

As an example of a typical situation, suppose a women's support group meets every Wednesday afternoon at Louise's house. This Wednesday they are discussing this book and what it might mean for them. Mary is allergic to wheat. Joanne is allergic to carrots. Louise, acting as Tester, uses Joanne as a Surrogate to test Mary. That is, Joanne touches Mary while Mary holds carrots on her abdomen. Joanne's arm tests strong because Mary is not allergic to carrots. When Mary holds wheat on her abdomen, Joanne's arm tests weak, showing that Mary is allergic to wheat. Now Louise tests Mary's arm while Joanne holds carrots, and Mary's arm tests weak because Joanne is allergic to carrots. When Joanne holds wheat, Mary's arm tests strong. Thus it is the allergy of the Subject who is being touched, not of the Surrogate, that is revealed through muscle testing on the Surrogate.

For best results in surrogate testing and correction procedures, some authorities believe that it is preferable for the Surrogate to be the same sex as the Subject. Emotional connections can also have important effects in surrogate testing. Because of the strong emotional attachment between parent and child, a parent generally is a good Surrogate for a child Subject. However, strong emotional effects between the Tester and the Surrogate can interfere with the testing process. That is, an emotional connection between the Subject and the Surrogate is not generally detrimental to accurate testing, whereas an emotional connection between Tester and Surrogate may interfere with the testing. In fact, if the Subject is experiencing a great deal of emotional turmoil, surrogate testing may be a good way to get past the emotional overlay in order to do accurate allergy and/or tolerance testing. If because of the emotional connection between husband and wife, or sister and brother, there is difficulty in testing, perhaps a neutral surrogate can provide an effective solution.

We have mentioned that you can use surrogate testing with your pets also. Test Spots and Tapping Spots on your dog, cat, or even bird are analogous to their location on humans. You may have a little more trouble if you have a pet snake; where, for example, are the snake's Underarm Test Spots? Fortunately, it is almost as effective to use the appropriate spots on the Surrogate as it is on the Subject.

Many deadly diseases such as kidney disease or feline leukemia are on the increase among household pets today. If we could determine more accurately whether our pets' diets are proper for them, we might be able to prevent much of this unnecessary illness. Surrogate testing is a way of finding out what our pets' allergies and tolerance levels are, and of improving upon the generally poor quality of commercial animal diets. Through surrogate testing we can determine what supplements our pets need to keep them at the peak of health.

Philip brought his elderly, sick cat to me to see if anything could be done. The cat had been diagnosed as having leukemia, but was already quite old. Through surrogate testing we were able to determine the cat's optimum feeding pattern and diet. We also determined some nutritional supplements the animal needed. Naturally we also tested for allergies and corrected them. That was more than five years ago. The cat is now well over 20 years old and going strong, with no sign of the leukemia. Without the surrogate testing probably nothing would have helped.

Please note: The preceding description does not mean that every case of feline leukemia is curable, or even that the methods I used "cured" the cat. There remains much scientific work to be completed before such conclusions could be drawn. This is only an anecdote, albeit a true one.

It may seem hard to believe, but you can even use surrogate testing to keep your plants healthy! Some people use surrogate techniques to determine whether their plants are getting enough water, the right kind of minerals or plant food, enough sun, etc. You may want to experiment with these techniques to see if they help you care for your plants. Perhaps reading Chapter 9, *Advanced Techniques for the Adventurous*, will help you get started.

Some of the ideas above may seem strange to you, but they do work. Give it a try—what have you got to lose?

6

Some Case Histories
Of Energy Work

Allergy can produce just about any symptom that humans are capable of experiencing. Because the Allergy Tap resolves the energy disturbances that underlie allergy, it can lead to the resolution of a wide range of problems. The case histories in this chapter represent my clinical experience with allergy problems over many years' time. Not all these cases were corrected with energy balancing techniques, since I have only been using these techniques for the past five years. However, in the earlier cases I did use muscle testing to identify the person's allergies, which we then dealt with through proper diet and supplements, and avoidance of the allergic substance.[11]

While allergy played a part in each of the problems described, simply correcting the allergy was not necessarily the only thing that needed to be done. For example, a proper nutritional program is another extremely important element in recovering from many physical and psychological disorders.

---

[11] Again, for a thorough description of these procedures, see *Energy, Allergy, and Your Health*.

Some of the "illnesses" illustrated in the following case histories are very common, nagging problems that bother many people. Others are less common, and may generally defy traditional treatment methods. When an underlying allergy is corrected in such cases, the results can be impressive and dramatic.

In cases where the Allergy Tap method will work, underlying energy disturbances are corrected virtually instantly. However, it may take some time for the body to repair the tissue damage which resulted from the allergy. In some of these case histories the person obtained immediate relief upon avoiding allergic substances or doing energy balancing, while in other cases it took some time, in addition to a more complex treatment program, to achieve recovery.

Remember, just because the examples below may have shown improvement does not mean that all such cases will do likewise. There may be a number of causes for any given "disease" and it is quite possible for allergy not to be involved at all. These are selected cases which may or may not be typical of other cases. Also, these energy techniques must not be considered as treatments for "disease"—they are only energy balancing methods. What response the body makes afterwards is up to it; the body does its own healing. Also, these are but a few of the tremendously wide range of possibilities. I firmly believe that allergies are involved in most so-called diseases. Keep in mind, however, that my definition of allergy is not the orthodox definition.

Recently I was in Bern, Switzerland, eating brunch with a friend from Germany. Alfred was eating a boiled egg. After a while I said, "I notice you are eating an egg."

"Yes."

"Well, do you remember three years ago when you attended my SET workshop? Do you remember what happened?"

He looked up, his mouth dropping slightly. "It is so easy for us to forget how things *were*. I had not remembered that until you reminded me now."

We reminisced. Alfred had been a participant in the Symbiotic Energy Transformation (SET) workshop, learning allergy testing and correction. He was terribly allergic to eggs, and moments after merely tasting one he began to wheeze, his face swelled, his eyes watered, and he looked miserable. We did the reflex points as quickly as possible, and the reaction began to subside. Just now he had eaten two eggs without even giving it a thought. Things had certainly changed.

Nasal Polyps

For years Arthur had suffered from asthma and nasal polyps. The polyps were so severe that he had to have them surgically removed every six months or so in order to breathe through his nose. After extensive allergy testing, we got Arthur off the foods to which he was sensitive and got him on a better diet, along with nutritional supplements. Within a few weeks the polyps that had been growing in his nose had begun reducing in size and finally disappeared entirely, so that Arthur could breathe normally through either nostril. His asthma was also getting progressively better. Arthur had been making continued progress over several months, with normal breathing, when he broke up with his girlfriend. Feeling depressed, he returned to eating the junk food we had carefully eliminated from his diet. With renewed exposure to allergic substances along with a poorer diet, Arthur's nasal polyps began to grow once again. He had no doubt at this point what he had to do to stay free of polyps.

Motion Sickness

Sometimes what appears to be motion sickness isn't that at all, but is an allergy. While Scuba diving, Jefferson got a dose of bad air containing some exhaust fumes from the boat's diesel engine which had been sucked into the air compressor. From that time on, whenever Jefferson went Scuba diving from a diesel-powered boat he would become "seasick," but under other conditions, or on a sailboat, he was perfectly all right. Sometimes it's not the motion, but rather chemical fumes within a vehicle—from faulty heaters, from exhaust fumes, or whatever—that can cause nausea and sickness.

Frequent Infections

Allergy can often lead to ear infections. When tissues swell as part of an allergic reaction, they can prevent fluids from draining down the eustachian tubes, allowing bacteria to become trapped, preventing toxins from draining out and nutrients from flowing in. This creates a situation where bacteria can grow readily. The following two cases show how allergies to a variety of foods can cause distressing ear infections in children.

Sean was only ten months old, and already he had had several ear infections. He had been given antibiotics on a number of occasions, but he still had chronic ear problems. His mother brought him in to my office, and allergy testing revealed that Sean was allergic to milk. When mother's milk and dairy products were eliminated from his diet, the ear infections stopped.

Molly also had frequent ear infections. Although ear infections are often related to dairy allergies, in Molly's case it was allergies to dust, hydrocarbons (petroleum chemicals), and molds that were causing her problem; dairy products were perfectly OK for her. Molly's parents cleaned out her room thoroughly, keeping out the dust and eliminating the molds. They changed the ventilation system which had been drawing fumes from the gas hot water heater into her room. In addition, we did the energy balancing techniques to eliminate Molly's allergies. Her ear infections were completely eliminated and have not recurred.

Colitis

Doreen was an attractive young woman in her early twenties who had been suffering from severe colitis for a number of years. Her symptoms included often severe diarrhea, gas, intestinal pains and cramps, and occasional bleeding. In addition she suffered from dehydration and low energy. Her condition was so bad by the time she came in to see me that her physician was urging her to have a large portion of her colon surgically removed, but so far she had resisted this suggestion.

We tested Doreen for allergies and changed her diet accordingly. Within only two weeks she was a new woman. Whereas previously she could barely drag herself in to my office, she now had abundant energy. Within a few months she was water skiing and leading the active life of a normal, healthy young woman. She has continued to avoid allergic foods for four years now, and her colitis problems have not returned.

Colon Polyps

Donald had experienced colon discomfort for some time. When he began to have occasional bleeding, he finally went in for a medical exam. Thorough medical evaluation revealed polyps growing in his descending colon. Some of these polyps were removed surgically, but they continued to grow back. In desperation Donald came to my office. We discovered that he was allergic to coffee, wheat, dairy products, and shellfish. After eliminating these from his diet, his bleeding disappeared and subsequent medical examination found no evidence of polyps.

Arthritis

Very often, when my clients see a dramatic improvement as a result of eliminating troublesome foods from their diet, they return to these foods prematurely. One of these people was Jessie, a woman who complained of a pain in her right knee and left shoulder. Among other things, she gave up eating wheat and related grains. Within a couple of weeks both her knee pain and her shoulder pain were gone. Since she was feeling so much better, she bought some sprouted wheat bread at a health food store, thinking that because the grain was sprouted it would be all right to eat it. She went home and ate a piece of the sprouted wheat bread and within a couple of hours her knee and shoulder pains had returned. When she told me what had happened I told her I was glad she had done what she did, because nothing I could have told her would have had more impact than her having had that experience. Now Jessie really understands what I mean when I say she must (temporarily) eliminate wheat (and the same-family grains of rye, barley, and oats) *completely* from her diet.

Because arthritis involves tissue damage, it may take a couple of weeks or more following the Allergy Tap treatment before the pain goes away. In this case it's not the allergic reaction that was producing the joint pain, but the damaged tissues. Once the allergic reaction has been taken care of, the tissue can begin to heal.

Muscle Tension

One of my friends had had muscle tension in her shoulders for years, so that she carried her shoulders unnaturally high. She explained this as psychological stress. I determined that the tension in one shoulder was due to a legume allergy, and when we used the Allergy Tap technique the shoulder on that side dropped dramatically—around one and one-half inches in a matter of ten minutes. Immediately afterwards she told me that she had never felt so relaxed in her life. I subsequently corrected a chemical allergy, which allowed the other shoulder to drop.

Premenstrual Syndrome (PMS)

Felice tended to become moody, irritable, forgetful, anxious, and depressed around her period, as well as experiencing food cravings. On allergy testing we found that she was allergic to soy, chemicals, chicken, and some pollens. When her allergies to these were corrected, along with a nutritional program, her psychological symptoms were relieved.

Fertility Problems

Louise came in to my office explaining that she had been told, both in Europe and in the United States, that she could never have children, presumably because of scar tissue in her fallopian tubes from previous pelvic inflammatory disease (PID).

Muscle testing revealed that it was not scar tissue that was a problem, but rather an allergic reaction to several foods which was causing swelling in the tubes and blocking the passageways. After identifying the foods, pollens, and molds to which Louise was allergic and correcting her allergies to these substances, the swelling went away. She is now the mother of two beautiful little girls, the products of two successful pregnancies.

Fibrocystic Breast Disease

Eileen was a certified acupuncturist who came to my office quite frightened. She had recently discovered a small lump in her breast, and had been even more frightened by her medical examination. Allergy testing revealed allergies to chemicals, cats, and several foods. After only ten weeks of eliminating these foods, and correcting the allergies, her breast lump was no longer detectable.

Gretchen had had a breast lump about the size of a golf ball for many months, and now it was beginning to grow, which was very upsetting for her. We did allergy testing and eliminated soy, the lactose fraction in milk, citrus, and tomatoes. In addition we did energy balancing to eliminate her allergies to molds and certain chemicals. Gradually the lump began to diminish in size. This took much longer in Gretchen's case because it was a much denser lump, but after about a year on a program of diet and supplementation, the lump is gone. Gretchen's case shows that allergy-based problems do not always clear up quickly. Larger, more heavily calcified or mineralized lumps may take longer for the body to dissolve.

Prostate Enlargement

Reggie was an active, high-spirited old gentleman in his 70s. One day he collapsed at his golf club. Fortunately, two physicians, fellow club members, were present and managed to keep him alive until he got to the hospital. Reggie was found to have massive heart failure, which led to triple bypass surgery. After he was released from the hospital, he reluctantly (he wasn't sure "all this stuff" would help) came to my office with his wife, who had been a client of mine for several years. Reggie told me that he wanted to enhance his healing rate from his surgery. He also disclosed that the doctors had found he had an enlarged prostate, and had recommended surgery as soon as he had recovered sufficiently from his cardiac problem. We did allergy testing and started Reggie on a program of avoiding certain foods, eating generally better, and taking nutritional supplements. After only three months his prostate was judged to be perfectly normal and surgery was no longer considered. (By the way, his heart is doing just fine.)

This case is interesting because many men are led to believe that prostate enlargement is an inevitable part of the aging process. In many cases, an enlarged prostate is partly allergic in origin, as well as due to deficiencies of certain nutrients. When these problems are resolved, prostate enlargement is sometimes corrected very easily.

Cancer

When Alan first came to me he had a medically documented case of lung cancer. After allergy testing he was placed on a nutritional program which went quite well until he eventually reached something of a plateau. At that time, muscle testing revealed he was having a reaction to the drug inhaler he was using for his asthma. We used energy balancing methods to change this reaction, and he immediately felt dramatically better. He spontaneously commented during the following session about how "that stuff we did last week" made him feel so different. After that he had dramatic improvement in the lung cancer, to the point that his x-rays shortly thereafter showed his lungs were totally clear. Three years later there has been no evidence of any cancer.

Miriam came in to me with a diagnosis of brain tumor. Because of her delicate health, we had to do the energy balancing procedures slowly, taking five separate sessions to get all the allergy corrections done. Within two weeks after completion of the allergy correction, Miriam's x-rays no longer showed any evidence of tumor, and she was able to take a long-postponed trip abroad.

People with cancer who receive nutritional support and allergy correction procedures often report that they are better able to tolerate any radiation and/or chemotherapy that they may undergo in addition. They tell me that their radiologists comment about how well they are tolerating radiation, and those receiving chemotherapy may not lose their hair. I believe that it is nutritional support that is the critical factor in helping people to avoid the uncomfortable side effects of radiation and chemotherapy.

* * * * *

Some very common problems are often related to allergy. Instead of giving numerous case histories below, I will discuss some of these problems in general terms, since they apply to so many people.

Addictions

I have observed over and over again that alcoholism and drug abuse often include significant allergic problems. Alcoholic beverages contain many substances that are not listed on the labels, to which some people can be highly allergic. Some of these substances are foods. For example, beer contains barley, corn, and hops, all of which can produce allergic reactions. Beer and wine also contain a large number of additives to which some people can be highly allergic. Hangover is generally not from the alcohol, but rather from these or other "contaminants." I believe that hangover is primarily an allergic and overload reaction to these substances.

Excess Weight and Eating Disorders

Food addictions. It is just as possible to become addicted to a food as it is to alcohol or narcotics or cigarettes. How does a food addiction become established? People may begin with no particular reaction to a given food, but then as their bodies begin to deteriorate they develop a sensitivity, or a lowered tolerance, to that food. Then, they can become actually allergic to the food. As the imbalance becomes greater, the body, in an effort to cope with this more severe imbalance, produces an addiction. It does not matter whether the addiction is to alcohol or heroin or coffee or milk or orange juice; it is the *body* which actually produces the addiction, not the substance to which it is addicted. Now if the person does not get his "fix"—a drink of alcohol, or of milk, for example—the body will go through withdrawal symptoms. Every time there is an addiction, there is an allergy. This has been recognized by progressive allergists for some time now.

Food addictions are sustained because people feel better when they get their "fix"; by drinking their milk or coffee they avoid their headache, weakness, or other symptoms. Some of my clients tell me, "I know milk is good for me because I feel so much better after I drink it." If they are addicted to milk, they may go through reactions such as craving and feeling out of control, which strongly resemble the withdrawal reactions from alcohol or other drugs. Since drinking the milk prevents any withdrawal reaction they feel better if they have their milk.

Psychological / Behavioral

One of the most important discoveries in the field of allergy has been the connection between food allergies and a wide range of psychological and behavioral problems. It is quite common, for example, that when people go on a fast their symptoms clear up, including their psychological symptoms. The Russians have done a great deal of work in this area. Over the past 25 years a Russian physician has used fasting to produce remarkable recoveries in thousands of mentally ill patients who did not respond to any other kind of treatment. The problem is how to maintain these recoveries when the fast is terminated, since when people return to eating once again, they are likely to consume foods to which they are allergic.

The recognition of allergic problems could potentially have a tremendous impact on our nation's crime rate and mental health. Authorities are increasingly acknowledging that dietary factors, including allergies and blood sugar reactions, may lie at the root of many mental and behavioral problems. Possible food allergies have been implicated in a wide range of criminal behavior, including violence, delinquency, stealing, and child abuse.

Among children today hyperkinetic behavior, or hyperactivity, is an increasing concern. The so-called Feingold Diet eliminates foods to which children are suspected to be unusually sensitive, including all food additives and foods containing salicylates. On this diet, many parents report vast improvements in their youngsters' behavior.

"Problem" Disorders

Autoimmune diseases. I personally believe that there is no such thing as autoimmune disease—that is, diseases in which the immune system for some mysterious reason begins to attack the tissues of the body it is supposed to defend. I have found in every case of a condition that is considered "autoimmune," that there has been an allergy to some substance or substances outside the body. When those allergies were corrected, the "autoimmune disease" began to improve or go away.

Many Factors Are Involved in Health Problems

Remember that the cases we have discussed in this chapter are all extremely individual. Because one person reacts to a certain food or chemical a certain way doesn't mean that someone else will react in the same way to the same thing. Moreover, there are multiple factors involved in most of these situations. It is not simply allergy that is causing the problems, but also nutritional and dietary imbalances, the person's general state of health, level of exercise, and psychological factors. In this book we are focusing on allergy-related issues, but usually there are other issues that must also be addressed in dealing with people's psychological and physical problems. There is more to being healthy than just doing the Allergy Tap. In addition to doing this process you may also require nutritional supplementation, psychological energy work, or other kinds of professional help.

Please note: Just as the previous chapter warned that these anecdotes are not claims or even evidence for the efficacy of these methods in the "treatment of disease," the same is even more true of the stories above. About the strongest claim which can be made about these cases is that they *may* indicate that allergies (as defined by this book), intolerances, and nutritional deficiencies might possibly have some relationship (not necessarily causative) to the conditions described. Years of properly carried out scientific research will be needed before any such claims can be made. On the other hand, since many of the conditions described above are considered "incurable," and since these techniques are seemingly harmless, I believe they should be tried. In Appendix G is a form with which you can report to me a summary of your experiences. These will be tabulated as a small part of the needed research.

7

Candida:
The Allergy Connection

The "Disease of the Decade"

Awareness of *Candida albicans* infections has become widespread during recent years.[12] Thanks to the publicity it received in such popular books as Dr. William Crook's *The Yeast Connection*, this fungus has become a very popular explanation for a wide variety of illnesses. Candida occurs in two forms. It enters the body as a yeast-like form, which under certain conditions may then convert into a fungus which can penetrate the mucosal linings of organs and invade the body, carrying toxic materials along with it. Thus Candida can infect the body in a variety of locations, with the symptoms it produces depending on where in the body the Candida is located. If it affects the skin, Candida can produce mysterious lesions and rashes or long-standing acne; if it takes up residence in the digestive tract it can produce indigestion, gas, and other forms of gastrointestinal distress; if it invades the nervous system it can produce fatigue, mood swings, and chronic headaches;

---

[12] It is estimated that over one third of the U.S. population has at least some Candida infection. Similar proportions are given for Europe, but England seems to be over 40%.

in the joints it can produce arthritis-like pains. I have seen one case where it caused alcoholism.

Many people experience such symptoms of long standing and may not be aware that their problem is due to Candida. Other people, influenced by the flood of publicity concerning Candida, and bewildered by their symptoms, are convinced that they have a Candida infection when in fact they do not.

Candida albicans is normally present in the human body, living in its yeast form in the intestinal tract. It is only when the yeast begins to proliferate and change to the fungus form that it begins to cause problems. Dr. Crook in his book attributes much of the problem with Candida to the prolonged use of antibiotics. Women who use oral contraceptives, according to Crook, are also more likely to develop an overgrowth of Candida. I believe the fundamental cause is weakening of the immune system due to nutritional deficiencies. These deficiencies are from our generally poor diet coupled with the body's increased need for nutrients to fight environmental toxins.

Anyone can develop a Candida infection. In young infants, colic is often the result of a Candida infection in the intestines. Thrush, an infection characterized by white spots in the mouth, is a form of Candida infection. A very disturbing recent finding is that the presence of Candida in the mucosa of the mouth is now considered by the U.S. Center for Disease Control as the *single best predictor* for the development of Acquired Immune Deficiency Syndrome (AIDS). This does *not* mean that the Candida overgrowth has caused AIDS, but only that when a person has a weakened immune system then Candida overgrowth is more likely to occur. The same applies to other possible infections, too.

Once Candida overgrowth has occurred, it is a difficult infection to get rid of. Traditional treatment usually relies on antifungal drugs such as Nystatin. Unfortunately, I have found that most people have a very low tolerance for these drugs; moreover, these medications may not be able to get to the Candida in certain locations in the body.

The Allergy Approach to Candida

In my work with people with Candida, I have found that the symptoms people get from Candida are primarily allergic symptoms. It is not the overgrowth of Candida itself that is causing their problems so much as the body's allergic reaction to the fungus. In fact, it is because of the allergy that the fungus is able to proliferate out of control in the first place. Because of the allergy, the immune system is repelled by the Candida and is not able to fight it. This interpretation is not inconsistent with the orthodox medical view that Candida is an "immunosuppressant agent." In the vast majority of cases, I have found that once the allergy to Candida has been eliminated, the related symptoms clear up quickly. With the allergy out of the way, the body's immune system (if it has the right materials—namely, the correct nutrients) is able to attack the Candida and destroy it quickly.

I believe that the best way to deal with Candida is not to attempt to destroy the organism with outside agents, which are toxic to the body by their nature, but rather to correct the allergy and give the body the nutritional support it needs to build up the immune system to counterattack the Candida organism. This is usually a simple process, using the techniques outlined in this book. First we test the person to see if there is a Candida allergy present. The allergy is then corrected using energy techniques. Finally we give nutritional supplements to help the body in its fight against the Candida.

Testing and Treating Yourself for Candida Allergy

In this book we have provided an order form for the Candida extract you will need to determine whether you are allergic to Candida.[13] To use these special papers, cut off a small piece, about 1/4 inch square, and use it for testing and correction procedures, as you would for any other substance. Place the small piece of Candida extract-treated paper on the Substance Placement Area and do the usual allergy test. If you are not weakened by this test, then it is unlikely that you have a Candida infection. If your indicator muscle is weakened with this test, then you are allergic to Candida, and you should proceed to the Allergy Tap Test to determine whether the

---

[13] These specially prepared HKPapers™ contain highly diluted extracts of many substances, including foods, pollens, chemicals, molds, animal dander and hair, dust, tobacco, etc. The *Candida albicans* paper is available separately.

Allergy Tap will work to correct your Candida allergy. You *cannot* get Candida from this special paper.

Remember that the presence of an allergy to Candida does not necessarily mean that you have a Candida *infection*. While it has been my experience that people who have a Candida infection are also allergic to Candida, muscle testing alone is not sufficient to diagnose Candida infection.

Unlike most other allergies, I have found that the Allergy Tap will only work for about 40 percent of people allergic to Candida. This probably relates to the severity of the Candida infection—mild infections are easier for the body to handle. If the Allergy Tap procedure does not work, it is necessary to use the "long method" which I call the Symbiotic Energy Transformation™ (SET) technique. This requires the help of a qualified professional; see Chapter 10 for suggestions about how to find such professional help. Don't delay. The body always gives high priority to getting rid of Candida.

If the Allergy Tap Test indicates that you are among the 40 percent who will be helped by the procedures in this book, place the square of Candida-treated HKPaper™ in your mouth[14] and go on to do the energy balancing procedures as for any other substance. Once you have performed the correction procedure, you can use another small piece of the specially treated paper to test whether the Candida allergy is still present. It will not be.

Helping Your Body Through the Healing Process

The body will work quickly to kill off the Candida once the appropriate energy balancing methods have been used. Usually some 50 percent of the Candida organisms will have died off within the first three weeks.[15] As the

---

[14] If you object to placing the Candida extract-treated HKPaper™ in your mouth, you can place the paper over the Substance Placement Area to do the correction. This is somewhat less sensitive, but may suffice in your case.

[15] Assuming that the proper nutritional supplements are being taken, to provide support for the immune system. Data are from an analysis of 55 recent cases.

Candida organisms break down, they release toxic substances into the system which can cause uncomfortable, sometimes quite severe reactions, especially for people with moderate to severe Candida infections, as indicated by the intensity of their symptoms. Some people report tingling sensations over large areas of their bodies; fatigue, low energy and an increased need for sleep, or sometimes insomnia; digestive disturbances; or many other varied symptoms. Depending on how poorly nourished the body is to begin with, and how severe the Candida infection, these symptoms may be negligible or very pronounced. Not everyone experiences symptoms of this kind, but it is a good idea to be warned of this possibility before you begin with your Candida treatment. Keep in mind that if the Allergy Tap method works for you, then you probably do not have a severe infection, and so should not be terribly concerned about possible healing reactions.

By providing nutritional support for your body in its fight against the Candida, you can help to reduce the severity of any symptoms that might appear, and speed the healing process. It is particularly important to support the functions of the pancreas, the spleen, and especially the liver. If possible get help from an experienced nutritional consultant (not necessarily a Registered Dietitian). Ask around in health food stores for suggestions, too. If you must work on your own, here are some general guidelines:[16]

—Take multiple digestive enzymes.

—Take zinc, vitamin B12, folic acid, vitamin C, and vitamin A.

—Take chlorophyll, preferably in the crude extract oil form.

—Take tissue extracts, especially of liver, pancreas, spleen, thymus, and adrenal.

—Do *not* take a lot of calcium while you have Candida, because it interferes with the body's killing off of the Candida.

You may want to ask a trusted professional for recommendations of specific brands of supplements. I find that among the best products available are

---

[16] Remember, you can test supplements and herbs for allergy and tolerance, too.

those made by Standard Process, which you may obtain through your professional practitioner.

—Herbal preparations can also help the healing process. Considered especially useful for Candida infections is Pau d'Arco (or Taheebo). Swedish bitters is also said to be helpful.

I have developed two herbal formulas which many people find helpful. Formula One is for the situation where the Candida allergy has been corrected. Formula Two is for the case when the Allergy Tap method will not work. The purpose of these formulas is not to attack the Candida as such, but rather to help support your body's immune system in its fight with the overgrowing Candida.

Remember that tissue repair always lags behind the correction of the allergy per se. Once the Candida organisms have been killed off, the debris remains in the body, and it takes the body a while to get rid of this material. Don't assume that your Candida infection is cleared up just because you have corrected the allergy; it will take some time for your body to eliminate the organisms and toxins, and for the tissues to repair themselves.

A Strong Immune System Is Your Best Defense Against Candida

Because of its presence in many people who go on to develop AIDS, Candida is increasingly being recognized as a serious health problem. In my work with people with AIDS, I have found that they usually have very severe cases of Candida. As their Candida levels drop, their condition also improves.

If your immune system is kept strong and healthy, you are not likely to be allergic to Candida, and you will therefore not develop an overgrowth of the organism. Thus your best insurance against this dangerous fungus is a sensible all-around program of proper diet, nutritional supplements, avoidance of overloading your system, and wise lifestyle choices including proper exercise and plenty of rest.[17] Avoid drugs and other toxic substances.

THE HERBAL FORMULAS

The herbal formulas shown indicate enough herbs to last for as long as most people need to take the mixture—60 days for Formula One and 120 days for Formula Two. This totals a lot of herbs, but only one-half ounce is used each day. There is no problem with brewing as much as a 10-day supply, but be sure to keep the extra in the refrigerator. If you wish to vary the flavor of the mixture (and have tested OK) you may add a little honey, or a small amount of mint, licorice root, vanilla bean, orange peel, hibiscus, or rose hips. These are added *after* the other herbs have been measured out to brew (in addition to the 1.5 ounces of the other herbs).

Formula One is used by people who have already had their Candida allergy corrected, while **Formula Two** is used by people whose Candida allergy has not been corrected.

---

[17] Not only are these topics discussed in the now oft mentioned *Energy, Allergy, and Your Health*, but also in another forthcoming book, *Dr. Scott's High-Calorie Weight Control Diet (and Program for Good Health)*.

HERBAL FORMULA ONE

Herb	Proportion
Black Cohosh	8 ounces
Coltsfoot	24 ounces
Cumin	8 ounces
Damiana	8 ounces
Dandelion	24 ounces
Goldenseal	16 ounces
Nettle	24 ounces
Wood Betony	8 ounces

Pulverize herbs in a blender. Pour 24 ounces of boiling spring water over 1.5 ounces of the mixture. Steep 15 minutes. Let cool, and drink 8 ounces three times a day, between meals. Continue for about 60 days.

* * * * * * * *

HERBAL FORMULA TWO

Herb	Proportion	Herb	Proportion
Black Cohosh	10 ounces	Burdock	10 ounces
Coltsfoot	30 ounces	Horsetail	20 ounces
Cumin	10 ounces	Lobelia	10 ounces
Damiana	10 ounces	Mugwort	20 ounces
Dandelion	30 ounces	Mullein	10 ounces
Goldenseal	20 ounces	Skullcap	10 ounces
Nettle	30 ounces		
Wood Betony	10 ounces		

Pulverize herbs in a blender. Pour 24 ounces of boiling spring water over 1.5 ounces of the mixture. Steep 15 minutes. Let cool, and drink 8 ounces three times a day, between meals. Continue for about 120 days.

8

Questions About The Energy Techniques

What if the allergy tap procedure won't work for me?

There are two reasons why the Allergy Tap method may not work. First of all, it may not work because you haven't done it correctly. Secondly, you may have followed the procedure correctly, but it just wasn't enough to correct your allergies. If on retesting you find your allergy has not been corrected, go back and repeat the entire process, making sure you have followed the instructions exactly. If you still don't get the expected results, wait a while before repeating, or try the process with another person acting as Tester. When the Allergy Tap procedure is properly done, for the cases in which testing shows that it will work (about 90 percent of cases), I have never yet seen a failure. If the Allergy Tap Test shows that the Allergy Tap will *not* work in your particular case, you will need to consult a qualified practitioner who is familiar with the more complicated Symbiotic Energy Transformation™ for correcting allergies.

Of course, sometimes the Allergy Tap method will not be appropriate for the Subject, or for the substance in question. In working with tolerances, for example, the Tolerance Tap procedure only works in 10 percent of cases anyway. Be sure that you properly perform the Tolerance Tap Test to see if tolerance can be increased for this Subject and for the substance in question.

What if I can't use the parts of the body described?

Suppose the Subject has an arm in a cast, or for some other reason cannot use an arm for muscle testing. One solution is to do surrogate testing, as described in Chapter 5. As long as some part of the Subject's body can be touched by the Surrogate, all allergy and tolerance testing can be done on the Surrogate instead of the Subject. Of course, this means that three people are involved in the procedure instead of only two.

However, you don't need to use a surrogate, since you can actually use just about any muscle in the body for testing, although some are easier to use than others. If for some reason you can't use the Subject's arm, you can try any other muscle. For example, you can use the quadriceps muscle in the leg; while the Subject holds the leg up with the knee bent, the Tester pushes down on the knee. Other leg muscles can be tested by having the Subject hold the outstretched legs together, while the Tester tries to pull them apart; or the Subject holds the legs out and the Tester tries to pull them inward. There are many other muscles that can be used for testing also. If you can't get any of those described to work for you, see Chapter 10 for suggestions about how to find help from a qualified practitioner.

Another problem that may arise is that some of the Tapping Spots cannot be used on the Subject. For example, an arm may be amputated, making the spots on the fingers unavailable; or a leg may be in a cast, making it impossible to tap the spots on the toes and feet. Or perhaps the Subject has a severe burn scar which obliterates a tapping spot.

In the case of amputations, the corresponding tapping spots will still be somewhere on the stump. However, finding the right spot is probably best done with the help of a knowledgeable professional. Where there is severe scarring or the tapping spots are otherwise inaccessible, you can generally use the closest spot on the same meridian as the tapping spot in question. Without expert help, however, you probably will not know the location of the appropriate meridian. One possibility is to try tapping all around the area, as close as you can get to the designated tapping spot.

Sometimes you may be able to tap the spots on one side of the body, but not on the other. In this case simply tap all the spots that are accessible, and then test to see if this procedure has been sufficient.

Many people find that it is effective to tap the Tapping Spots on a Surrogate while the Surrogate is touching the Subject. You may want to give this a try to see if it will work for you.

Whatever method you use when you are not able to tap certain spots, be sure to retest the Subject afterwards, and you may well find that the allergy has been eliminated.

What if I just can't find what I am allergic to?

If you believe you are still allergic to something which you just cannot identify, there is a possibility you can still correct the unknown allergy. The first step is to correct every other allergy you can. Then collect a few drops of your own fresh urine in a cup. If you do test allergic to the urine then you have confirmed that, indeed, you still have an allergy to some substance to which you are currently being exposed. Test to see whether this allergy is correctable. If so, then do the corrections. If not, the best solution is to get help from a professional who knows the SET technique (see Chapter 10). This urine test works because residues will be produced from any allergic substance that enters your body. Remember, however, the earlier discussion about using substances in as simple a form as possible. Too many allergic substances together will not be correctable with the quick Allergy Tap method. Note that testing your own urine may reveal the existence of allergies that you did not suspect.

Is this just a placebo effect?

No. There are good reasons to believe that the changes that occur in a person who has undergone the Allergy Tap procedure are not from placebo or suggestion effects. If you were to ask any of the people whose case histories have been given in this book, they would state with certainty that it is not merely a placebo. Generally these people had already tried many different approaches without obtaining relief, until finally the Allergy Tap method worked for them.

In some cases clients have come to me with the results of other allergy tests, such as blood tests, that were done previously. After doing the energy work, these blood tests when repeated showed a change in reactivity.

Further evidence that this method is not just a placebo comes from its success in working with infants and animals. For example, I used the Allergy Tap with a six-week-old nursing infant who was allergic to wheat that the mother was eating. After we did the energy technique on the baby, he no longer reacted to the wheat in his mother's diet. It is unlikely that a six-week-old infant could react to this sort of placebo, but if he could, then by all means let's make use of it! Our goal is to get people functioning better.

Of course the best evidence for the reality of the Allergy Tap method is whether it works for you. If it does, then you can decide for yourself whether it is just a placebo.

Well, if this is not a placebo, is it suggestion or some other psychological response?

These effects definitely are not suggestion or hypnosis. Again, infants or animals would not respond so readily if this were the case. On the other hand, I do consider that these effects are psychological in nature. For several reasons, much too complex to describe in this book,[18] I believe that the energy system is ultimately controlled by our brain/mind. Indeed, allergies can also be corrected through certain psychological methods, though not as efficiently as with these procedures.

How long will it take to see the effects of this process?

In terms of changes in the body's energy, the effect occurs immediately. However, if the energy disturbances in your body have produced physical changes, or tissue reactions, it may take a while for the tissues to heal to the point where you can actually feel the difference.

Some of the best evidence for the effectiveness of the Allergy Tap is the great speed with which things happen after the technique has been used.

---

[18] *Energy, Allergy, and Your Health,* however, does discuss these concepts in some detail, as will some of the other books in this series.

Often, as soon as we correct an allergy to a certain substance the individual clearly begins to experience an improvement in symptoms. For example, in the case of the art student mentioned in Chapter 2, as soon as we used the Allergy Tap procedure, she was immediately able to go to school without getting headaches. Similarly, in the case of the woman who carried her shoulders high because of allergy-based muscle tension (see Chapter 6), the shoulder actually went down while were doing the energy procedure.

On the other hand, in the case of an arthritic joint, or swollen, inflamed membranes in the respiratory tract, it may take a while for the body to clear the damaged tissues and for the pain to go away. Depending on the tissues involved and the severity of the involvement, it may take hours, days, or even weeks for improvement to be noticed. Support from diet improvement or nutritional supplements may also be required to achieve best results.

We must also warn that even though you may correct your allergy you must still be careful to keep your intake of the substance in question below your tolerance level, as we have explained in Chapter 4. Also, remember that allergy alone is rarely the sole cause of some problem. Other lifestyle changes may need to be accomplished.

How long will the treatment hold?

The Allergy Tap treatment holds indefinitely. I have retested people after more than three years, with no deterioration in their condition. I cannot say at this point that the treatment holds forever, because I have only been using these techniques for about four years; but I have not yet seen a single case in which the allergy has returned. The SET procedure has been used since 1981, with no example of returned allergy. Be sure not to confuse overloading (exceeding tolerance level) reactions with allergic reactions.

For example, one woman had a pain in the side of her neck every time she ate almonds. She never got this pain unless she ate almonds, and she got it every time she ate them. On testing she was indeed found to be allergic to almonds, so we did the SET energy balancing procedure to correct her almond allergy. We then tested her *tolerance* for almonds, and found she could eat 26 almonds or less without harm. She went home immediately and ate 26 almonds without getting any reaction. It has been five years now, and she still doesn't get any reaction from eating almonds below her tolerance level.

What is the Symbiotic Energy Transformation™ (SET) method?

SET is the method of allergy correction which preceded the Allergy Tap procedure described in this book. Although the energy system and energy reflex points are utilized by the SET method, the actual process is more complex. Since the SET method is also considerably more powerful (apparently 100% effective), it is being taught only to selected qualified professionals. See Chapter 10 for more information about how to find one of these professionals, should the Allergy Tap not be adequate for your needs.

9

Advanced Techniques For The Adventurous

Asking Your Body Questions

After you have used the allergy and tolerance procedures for a while, you may want to explore how you can tap even further into your body's energy system. Using muscle testing to "ask your body questions," you enable your body to tell you where you are experiencing energy disturbances, and why.

Actually, you have already been using energy techniques to ask your body questions. You have observed that an indicator muscle tests strong when you say "Yes" or your true name, but becomes weak when you say "No" or give a false name. Now that you have had some practice using muscle testing in allergy work, you can extend these techniques even further.

These advanced techniques will help you do a much more thorough job of identifying and correcting allergies and intolerances. However, you must be very careful to ask questions properly, or you will get misleading answers.

Begin with the simple procedures you already know. First make sure that the Subject's indicator muscle tests strong, properly balancing it if necessary. Then have the Subject say "Yes." Muscle testing should show the arm to be strong. Now have the Subject say "No." The arm should now test weak. Have the Subject say, "My name is . . . [correct name]." The arm should test strong. When the Subject says, "My name is . . . [false name]," the arm should test weak. If these preliminary tests do not produce the expected results, refer back to the section on muscle testing in Chapter 1, or to Appendix A, and follow the procedures for balancing the muscle.

Now that the indicator muscle is strong and balanced, you can proceed to ask the Subject's body a series of questions related to allergies and intolerances. For all these questions, if the muscle tests *strong* it is a "Yes" response, and if it tests *weak* the response is a "No."

Be sure to intersperse "blank" questions from time to time, (such as, "Is Subject's name [true name]?"), to make sure that the indicator muscle is still responding correctly.

Sample Questions About Allergy

1. Have at least some of my allergies been corrected?

2. Have all of my allergies been corrected?

Note that we distinguish between *some* and *all*; this is the kind of logic that must be observed when asking questions with muscle testing. In other words, asking the ambiguous question "Have my allergies been corrected?" may not produce a useful response.

If muscle testing reveals that not all allergies have been corrected, perhaps you can find out what category the remaining allergies are in.

3. Do I still have any FOOD allergies?

4. Do I still have any POLLEN allergies?

5. Do I still have any CHEMICAL allergies?

6. Do I still have any ANIMAL allergies? . . and so on.

Using this technique, you can also check to see whether a certain symptom you have been experiencing—that itchy rash, that dripping nose, that arthritic joint—might be related to allergy. Remember, once again, that it is very important that you phrase your questions correctly. You might begin as follows:

7. Is SYMPTOM XYZ *at least partly* related to allergy?

Here it is possible to get into logical difficulties. Perhaps your allergies have already been corrected through the energy techniques you learned from this book. Then whatever remains of the symptoms would be due to some other cause, and the correct answer would be "No." The arm muscle would then test weak. If all your allergies have been corrected, you should then phrase the question, "*Was* SYMPTOM XYZ at least partly related to allergy?"

A follow-up question, if you receive a Yes answer to the either form of the preceding one, is:

8. Are there any more allergies to correct in order to help my body get rid of Symptom XYZ?

Sample Questions About Tolerances

You can ask similar questions about your body's tolerances for various substances. For example:

9. Are there any FOODS for which the Tolerance Tap Method will work?

10. Are there any POLLENS for which the Tolerance Tap Method will work?

11. Are there any CHEMICALS. . . etc?

As with allergies, you can ask whether specific symptoms are related to intolerances:

12. Is [or was] Symptom XYZ at least partly related to an intolerance?

13. Is the fact that I . . . [e.g., drink a half gallon of milk a day] related to Symptom XYZ?

You can also check to see whether certain elements of your diet are OK for you, or whether certain combinations are OK:

14. Is it OK for me to eat food XYZ right now?

15. How much? One cup? One-half cup? One tablespoonful? One-quarter teaspoonful? . . . etc?

16. Is it OK for me to eat food ABC with food XYZ? If so, how much? One cup? . . . etc.

17. How much total food should I eat now? One ounce of food? Two ounces? Two and 3/4 ounces? . . . etc.

18. Should I drink liquid QRS with food XYZ?

As you can see, there are virtually unlimited possibilities for tapping into your body's inner wisdom through muscle testing. Go ahead and experiment; have fun, and see what kinds of answers you get. Remember, though, that it is very easy to get tripped up because the questions must be absolutely precise and clear, and sometimes it's not easy to recognize that you are asking a question in an ambiguous way.

Psychological Factors and Allergy

The same kind of process can be extended to include psychological factors that may be contributing to your symptoms. You could ask, for example:

19. Is there anything else besides allergy related to Symptom XYZ? (This would be an appropriate follow-up to Questions #7 and #8.)

20. Is this factor psychological? Is it related to exercise? Is it related to diet?. . .etc.

Psychological factors are often deeply involved in allergies. The body gets set up for developing allergies by psychological processes that usually occur when we are very young. By dealing with the psychological processes properly, we can get rid of the allergies that arose from them. This doesn't mean that the psychological issue itself has been resolved—only that the allergy that resulted from it has been corrected.

Just as you have seen that exposure to certain physical substances can disturb your body's energy (as evidenced by weakening of the arm muscle), so can psychological factors disturb your energy. It is beyond the scope of this book to discuss how to resolve such psychological issues, but at this point you may want to observe for yourself how psychological factors interact with your body's energy system. The following "extra-advanced" techniques will give you an idea of how muscle testing can be used to explore this area.

Asking Questions About Psychological Processes

Have the Subject place one hand over the navel. Either hand may be used. (The navel is covered because all the acupuncture meridians have reflex points around the navel.) Use the other arm for muscle testing. Make sure that the arm muscle is properly balanced. Now have the person think about each of the following subjects, one at a time, as you name them:

—anger
—emotional intimacy
—success, failure
—dependence, independence

To be more specific have the person think, or say aloud, things such as:

I like my work.
I want to succeed as a composer (or whatever).
I must be dependent on my husband.
I want to marry "Jill."
I want to lose weight.

Have the Subject think about any particularly stressful situations—such as their relationship with their spouse, their children, their boss, their job, or their mother-in-law.

Not every one of these topics will weaken every person, but many people are weakened by at least some of them. This doesn't mean that they are neurotic or sick or crazy; it simply means that their energy is disturbed when these issues arise, which makes it more difficult to deal with them. These are stressful issues.

As you observe how simply thinking about certain issues can weaken your body's energy, you will understand that correcting allergies alone is not going to cure all your symptoms. Many psychological problems will improve when allergies are corrected, but other processes besides allergy underlie many problems also.

In a forthcoming book, *Relieve Your Own Emotional Distress and Phobias in Minutes,* I will go into greater detail about the psychological factors that weaken the body's energy, and will describe some techniques for correcting these problems. Your body's energy system is very fundamental to all aspects of your life. You can learn to work with this energy to help yourself, rather than having to rely on highly paid professionals who are often unable to help you.

One difficult area where energy techniques are helpful is dyslexia and other learning disabilities. Often these problems are the result of energy disturbances that can be corrected through energy techniques. Some of these techniques will be described in another forthcoming book in this series, *Improve Your Own Intellectual Functioning and Creativity in Minutes.*[19]

Energy Techniques for Breaking Harmful Patterns

We said earlier that the stage is set for the development of allergies on the basis of psychological events, especially those that happen early in childhood. These early psychological events cause us to develop certain patterns of functioning, ways in which we interact with our world. They set the stage not only for allergies, but also for how we deal with anger, intimacy, success and failure, and other issues in our lives. The energy techniques I have been describing are ways to break those patterns. When you break the pattern that originally set up the allergy, you don't have the allergy anymore. There are also ways to break the patterns that lead to other difficulties. For example, many people in our society have harmful patterns such as:

—binge eating
—smoking
—drinking too much
—relationship problems

---

[19] See Appendix G to learn how you can receive announcements for each of these books, and others, as they are released.

—job problems
—being depressed
—feeling angry
—feeling "stuck"
—drug use
—poor self-esteem
—self-sabotage
—and hundreds more

Such patterns underlie any situation where you find yourself doing something repetitively that is not in your best interest. When one of these patterns gets triggered, you deal with things, often inappropriately, according to that pattern. One of my favorite examples is what I call the "I'll never do it again" syndrome. You may engage in a self-destructive behavior —such as eating three candy bars in one sitting, drinking too much, or losing your temper with your spouse—and after you have gone through the whole thing you say, "I'll never do that again!" Yet when the same circumstance arises again, because your energy is disturbed, you are no longer in control, and off you go again in your undesirable behavior pattern.

You can ask your body questions to determine the source of these behavior patterns. For example, perhaps you have a harmful pattern of binge eating. Using muscle testing, you can ask your body such questions as:

21. Is (or was) my binge eating at least partly related to allergies/intolerances? (Note: If you have gotten this far in this book, most of your allergies should have been corrected by now.)

22. Is my binge eating at least partly related to psychological processes?

23. Is my binge eating at least partly related to nutritional deficiencies?

Which vitamins? A? E? etc.
Which minerals? Calcium? Zinc? Iron? etc.
Protein?

What can I eat to supply these?
Eggs? -raw? -cooked?
Spinach? -raw? -cooked?

Take pills? Which brand?
How many? 1 a day? 2 a day? etc.

This should give you an idea of how to proceed.

When you are stuck in a pattern, you have lost your control over the situation. There are methods available to deal with these repetitive, harmful patterns. These methods are known collectively as Health Kinesiology, and subsequent books in this series will describe some of the methods that you can learn to use yourself to help to correct the energy imbalances underlying these patterns and regain your control.

The purpose of this chapter is to give you ideas, not to give you complete procedures. Explore, have fun, and be careful not to blindly accept whatever you find. Muscle testing does have its limitations, so don't attempt to go too far without some training with a more experienced person. Don't place too much faith in the results until you have proven to yourself their accuracy with known situations.

10

How To Find Help
With The
Energy Techniques

This book is designed to teach anyone, regardless of their previous experience, to use muscle testing and energy techniques to resolve their allergy and intolerance problems. We have tried to anticipate all the questions that may arise, and to give clear, simple instructions about how to deal with them. However, you may have difficulty understanding certain instructions, or getting the Subject properly balanced, or even locating a point on the body.

Where can you find help if you encounter such difficulties? In this section we will give some suggestions about what kinds of professionals and non-professionals may be able to help you solve your problems in working with this book.

Sometimes valuable help can be obtained from laypeople. For example, you may have a friend or neighbor who has taken the basic Touch for Health class, as sponsored by the worldwide Touch for Health Foundation. Touch for Health is designed for laypeople. People trained in Touch for Health are likely to have reference materials that may be useful; or, because they are familiar with energy techniques, they may be able to help you understand the instructions in this book. If you inquire further, you will probably be able to find someone who is a Touch for Health instructor. Show this book to that person and they should be able to help you with your problem.

Other muscle testing systems, besides Touch for Health, include:

- applied kinesiology
- applied physiology
- behavioral kinesiology
- biokinesiology
- clinical kinesiology
- educational kinesiology
- hyperton-x
- kinesionics
- Health Kinesiology

People who practice any of these disciplines should be able to help you with problems you might encounter in working with this book. Because of the growing popularity of kinesiology, numerous varieties have been developing. Not all can be listed here.

Many people who have studied massage—either traditional massage or forms such as Shiatsu—have studied the body's energy system and may be able to help. Of course, acupuncturists and acupressurists are also familiar with the concept of body energy. Even if some of these practitioners are not familiar with muscle testing and associated energy balancing techniques, they should be able to help you locate reflex points or understand the instructions.

Chiropractors are another group of professionals who often study applied kinesiology, Touch for Health, or acupuncture. Naturopaths may also be familiar with energy techniques. Some psychologists are also familiar with these methods. If you need to locate a professional who understands energy techniques, look for chiropractors, psychologists, naturopaths, or others who work with applied kinesiology, or who advertise that they are concerned with allergy or nutrition-related work. Professional affiliations might include The International College of Applied Kinesiology (largely chiropractors) or the newer International Association of Specialized Kinesiologies.

Of course it would be ideal for an appropriate practitioner in your area to learn the techniques of Health Kinesiology. Holistically oriented health practitioners are more likely to be aware of these energy techniques, so you might ask one whom you particularly like to contact the Health Kinesiology Institute for information about training programs.

Finally, if all else fails, write to the Health Kinesiology Institute yourself. We may not be able to answer every letter personally, but we will do our best to let you know about the health professionals closest to your area who have learned these energy techniques through Health Kinesiology training programs.

We also urge you to report to us about your experience working with this book. If you notice changes in your symptoms—especially in such difficult problems as tumors, autoimmune diseases, etc.—please use the form in Appendix G to report on your results. The more evidence we can accumulate that these energy techniques work to eliminate allergies and the many problems allergy can cause, the easier it will be to perform additional research to develop and demonstrate the validity of this work.

Should you have any suggestions to improve future editions of this book, please let us hear from you. We will greatly appreciate it even if we are unable to answer every person individually.

ILLUSTRATIONS

Illustrations

All the illustrations have been placed together in this section to make it easier to find whichever one you need. Whether you are following the directions in the text itself or in the Appendices, you can use this convenient section to find or confirm the location of all energy reflex points.

Along the edge of each page you will note "tabs" which are either solid black or gray and which contain the Illustration numbers. These tabs are to help you find any Illustration quickly. The solid tabs indicate the principal reflex points and procedures, while the gray show those which are used less often.

To further assist you in relating the Illustrations to the text, at the end of each caption are the page numbers in the book where reference is made to that Illustration.

Once you have become familiar with the energy procedures, you should be able to use only the Short Version of the complete procedures as described in Appendix B, or the Flowchart, also found in Appendix B, along with these Illustrations.

Note that most of the reflex points are bilateral. That is, they appear symmetrically on both sides of the body even though many of the Illustrations show the point on only one side. The text makes clear reference (R&L, right and left) to each of these, and also specifies a few instances when the points occur on only one side of the body.

Illustrations

SECTION 1

Energy Balancing & Muscle Testing

SECTION 2

Allergy Testing & Allergy Tap

SECTION 3

Tolerance Testing & Tolerance Tap

SECTION 1

Energy Balancing & Muscle Testing

1

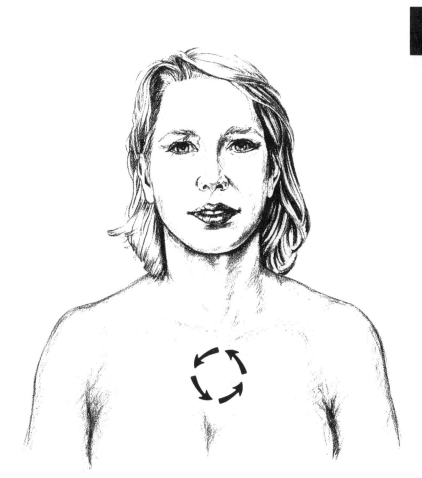

Illustration 1. Energy Balancing Spot, Area #1.
About two inches above the **v** where breastbone and collarbone meet, there should be a small bump, at the point where the 2nd ribs attach to the breastbone (sternum). This is the Energy Balancing Spot, or EBS (pp. 11, 141, 158).

Balancing Tap.
Tester (or Subject) taps around a circle 3" in diameter, centering around the EBS. Tap in a counterclockwise direction as Tester faces Subject. Tap for about 30 seconds, about 100 taps, using 1 or 2 fingers (pp. 11, 141, 158).

2A

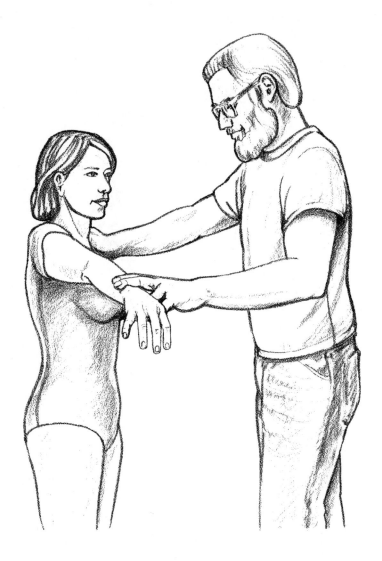

Illustration 2A. Muscle Testing, Standing Position.
Subject stands relaxed, with feet slightly apart. Subject holds out one arm with palm
facing down, holding it about 45 degrees off to the side, and about 45 degrees up (pp.
11, 142, 145).

2B

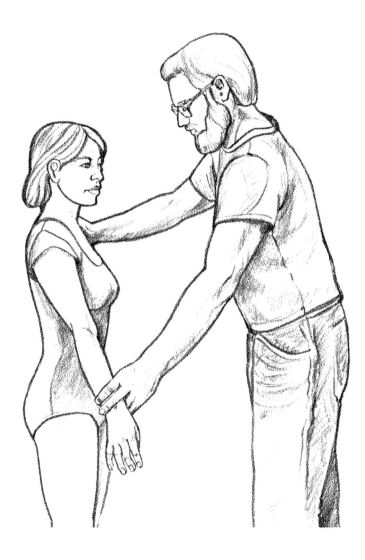

Illustration 2B. Muscle Testing Procedure.
With one hand on Subject's shoulder and the other hand on Subject's extended forearm, Tester presses down on the arm slightly above the wrist, while Subject tries to hold it straight. If indicator muscle is strong, Subject will be able to keep the arm raised. If it is weak, Subject's arm will give way (pp. 12, 142, 145).

3AB

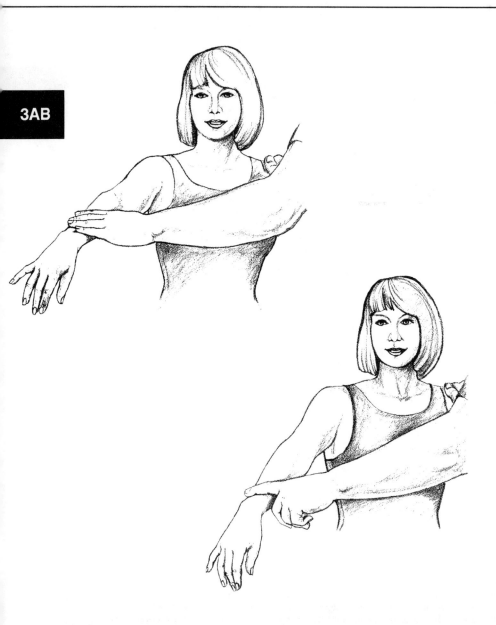

Illustrations 3A & 3B. Muscle Testing: Tester's Hand Position.
Tester presses on Subject's forearm with the palm or with four fingers, as shown in Illustration 3A. Only one or two fingers may be needed if Subject is weak, as shown in Illustration 3B (pp. 11, 142).

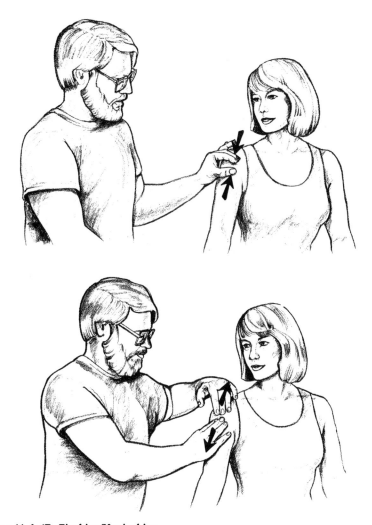

4AB

Illustrations 4A & 4B. Pinching/Unpinching.
A simple muscle test to see if indicator muscle is indicating properly.

Pinching: Broadly and gently pinch the muscle along side of upper arm, one or two inches below top of shoulder (Illustration 4A).   On muscle testing, the arm should test weak after this pinching procedure.

Unpinching: Use two hands, moving the fingers apart over the muscle rather than squeezing together (Illustration 4B).   Repeat muscle testing; indicator muscle should now test strong (pp. 13, 143).

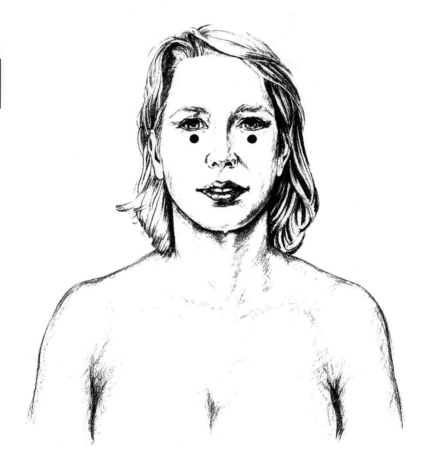

Illustration 5A. Spots #2 R&L.
These spots are located on the right and left cheekbones, just below the center of the eye. Used in Special Energy Balancing Procedure, Allergy Tap and Tolerance Tap (pp. 14, 34, 47, 143, 150, 156, 159, 161).

5BC

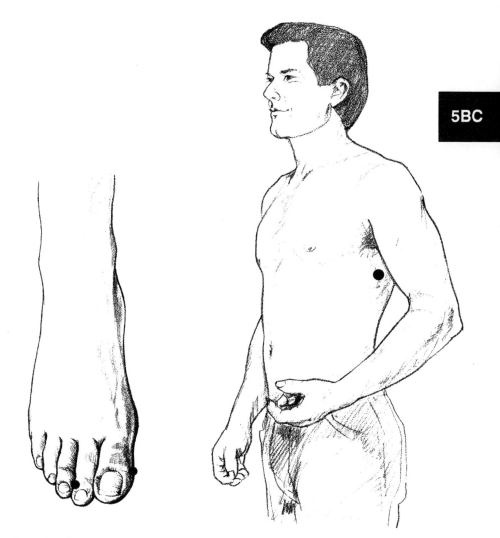

Illustration 5B. Spots #3 R&L.
Located on outer edge of right and left 2nd toe, just below the nail. Used in Special Energy Balancing Procedure, Allergy Tap and Tolerance Tap (pp. 14, 34, 47, 143, 150, 156, 159, 161).

Spots #5 R&L. Located on inner edge of right and left big toe, just below the nail. Used in Special Energy Balancing Procedure, Allergy Tap and Tolerance Tap; also as auxiliary Tolerance Tap Test Spots (pp. 14, 34, 45, 47, 143, 151, 154, 156, 159, 161).

Illustration 5C. Spots #4 R&L.
Located on right and left side, at a level halfway between crease of elbow and armpit. Used in Special Energy Balancing Procedure, Allergy Tap, Tolerance Tap Test and Tolerance Tap (pp. 14, 34, 47, 143, 151, 156, 159, 161).

6A

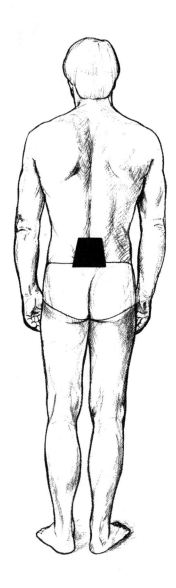

Illustration 6A. Area #6.
Located on mid lower back at belt level. Used in Special Energy Balancing Procedure
(pp. 14, 144).

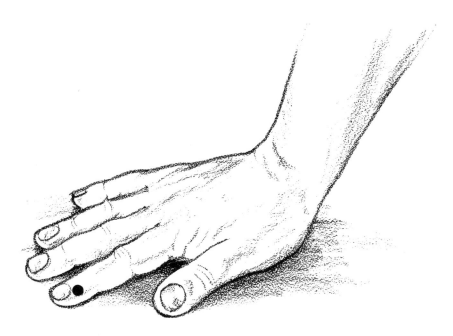

6B

Illustration 6B. Spots #7 R&L.
Located on inside edge of right and left index finger, at base of nail. Used in Special
Energy Balancing Procedure (pp. 14, 144).

7A

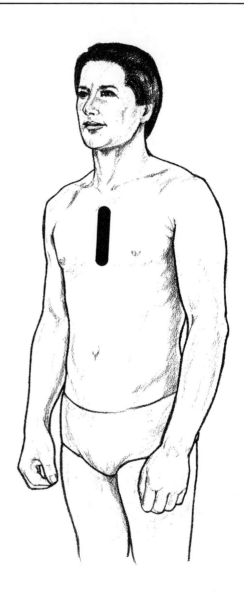

Illustration 7A. Area #8.
Located along center of breastbone. Used in Special Energy Balancing Procedure (pp. 14, 144).

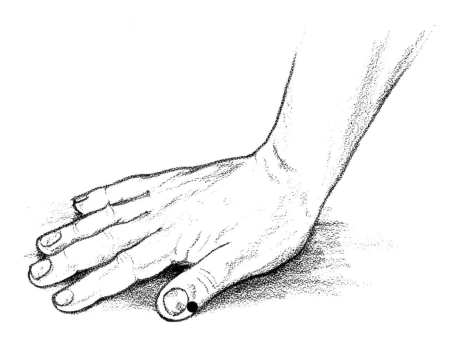

7B

Illustration 7B. Spots #9 R&L.
Located on side of thumb away from fingers, at base of nail. Used in Special Energy
Balancing Procedure (pp. 14, 144).

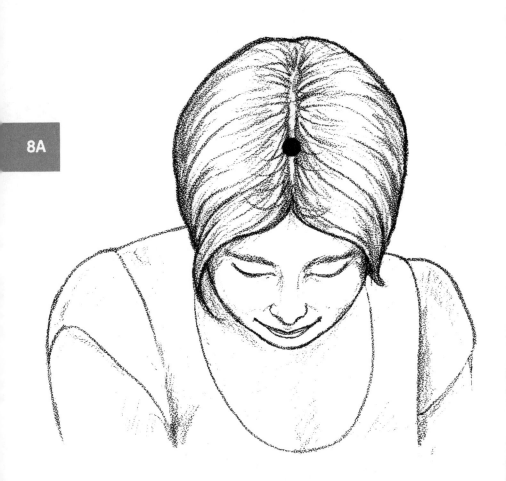

8A

Illustration 8A. Spot #10.
Located on top of skull. Used in Special Energy Balancing Procedure (pp. 14, 144).

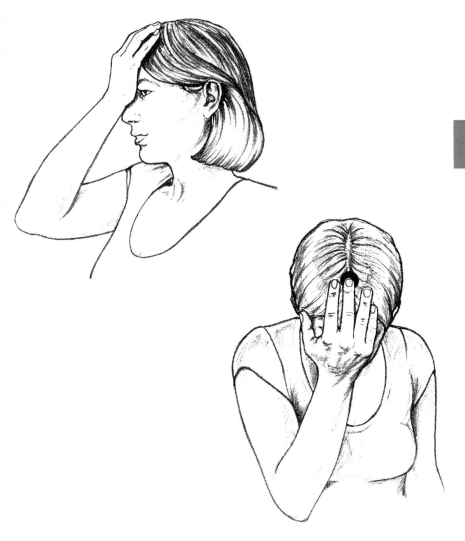

8BC

Illustrations 8B & 8C. Locating Spot #10.
Place palm on bridge of nose. Spot #10 will be at end of middle finger, on the top of the head (pp. 14, 144).

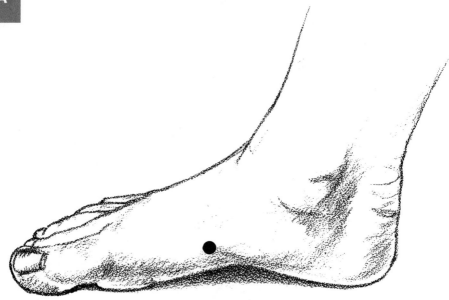

9A

Illustration 9A. Spots #11 R&L.
Located on inside edge of right and left foot, 1/3 distance between ball of foot and back
of heel. Used in Special Balancing Procedure if Subject tests weak when Tester alternates testing hand after Special Energy Balancing Procedure (pp. 15, 144).

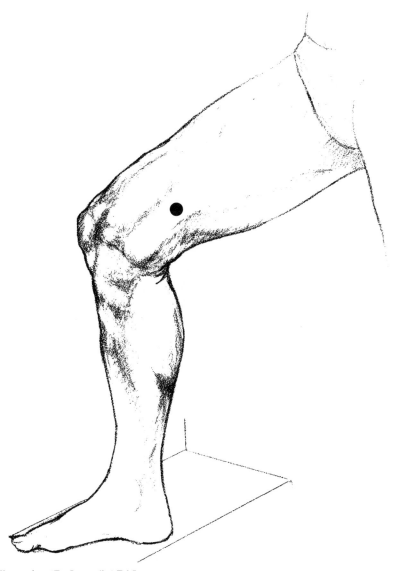

9B

Illustration 9B. Spots #12 R&L.
Located on inside upper leg, right and left leg, 1/4 distance between knee and crotch. Used in Special Balancing Procedure if Subject tests weak when Tester alternates testing hand (pp. 15, 144).

10A

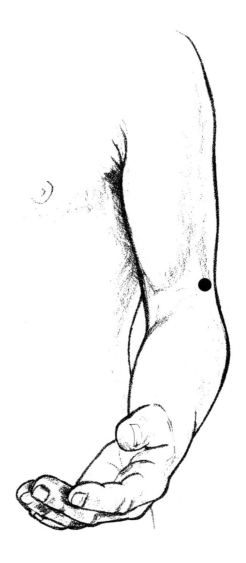

Illustration 10A. Spots #13 R&L.
Located just above crook of elbow, on outside edge of right and left arm. Used in
Special Balancing Procedure if Subject tests weak when Tester alternates testing hand
(pp. 15, 144).

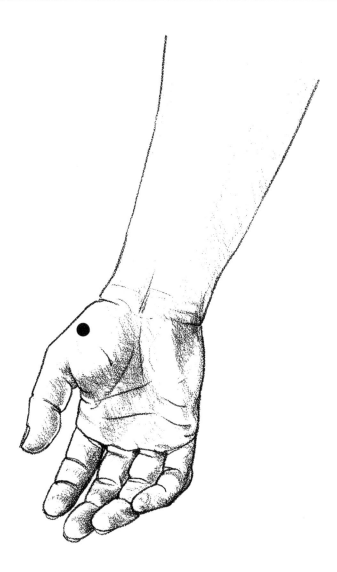

10B

Illustration 10B. Spots #14R&L.
Located on base of thumb, outside edge, center of fleshy part. Used in Special Balancing Procedure if Subject tests weak when Tester alternates testing hand (pp. 15, 144).

Allergy Testing & Allergy Tap

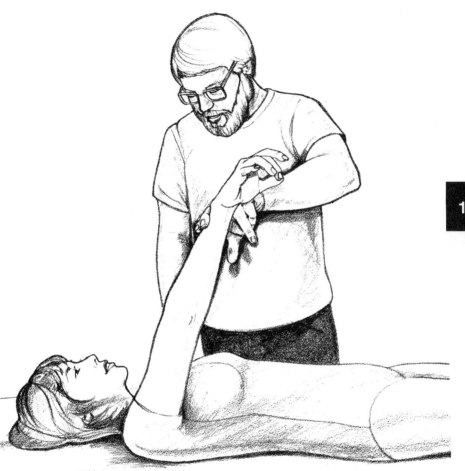

Illustration 11. Muscle Testing, Lying Position.
This is the most convenient position for allergy work. Subject holds arm straight up from body at angle of 30-60 degrees. Tester presses down on extended arm (pp. 16, 145).

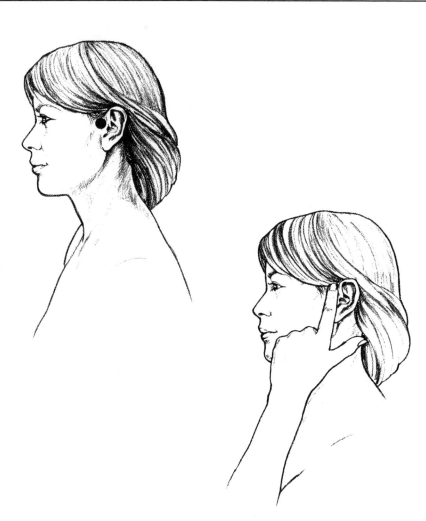

12AB

Illustration 12A. Allergy Test Spots, #15 R&L.
Located in front of right and left ear. Only one spot needs to be touched at a time. Used in Allergy Testing and procedure for strengthening indicator muscle if it is weakened by touching Allergy Test Spot (pp. 17, 18, 147, 158).

Illustration 12B. Locating Allergy Test Spot.
To be sure you are touching Allergy Test Spot, place finger along front of ear. Touch the spot lightly, and only while muscle testing is being performed (pp. 17, 18, 147, 158).

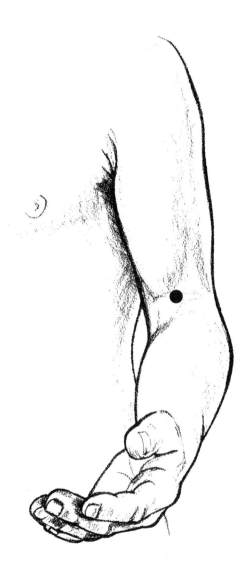

Illustration 13. Muscle Strengthening Spots, #16 R&L.
Located just above crease of elbow on right and left upper arm. Used to strengthen
indicator muscle if it tests weak simply from touching Allergy Test Spot (pp. 18, 147).

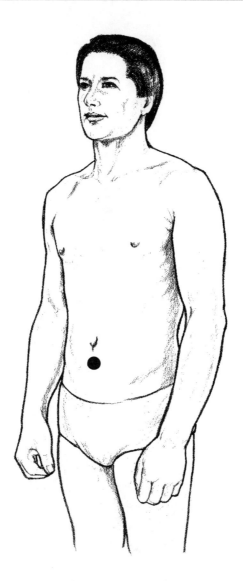

14A

Illustration 14A. Substance Placement Area (SPA), Area #17.
Located on abdomen, just below the navel. This is the area where test substances are
placed in Allergy Testing, Allergy Tap, Tolerance Testing and Tolerance Tap (pp. 18, 44,
148, 153, 155, 159).

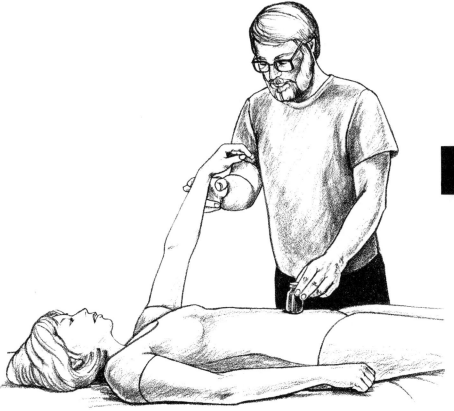

14B

Illustration 14B. Allergy Testing, Lying Position.
Test substance is in place on Substance Placement Area. Subject or Tester next touches
Allergy Test Spot while Tester tests indicator muscle (pp. 18, 44, 148, 159).

15A

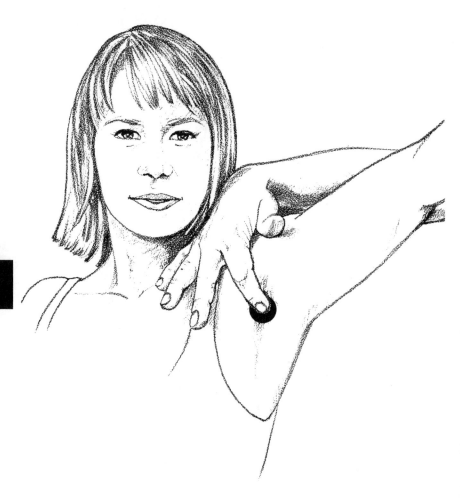

Illustration 15A. Allergy Tap Underarm Test Spots, #18R&L.
Located in right and left armpit. Used in Allergy Tap Test (pp. 29, 149, 159).

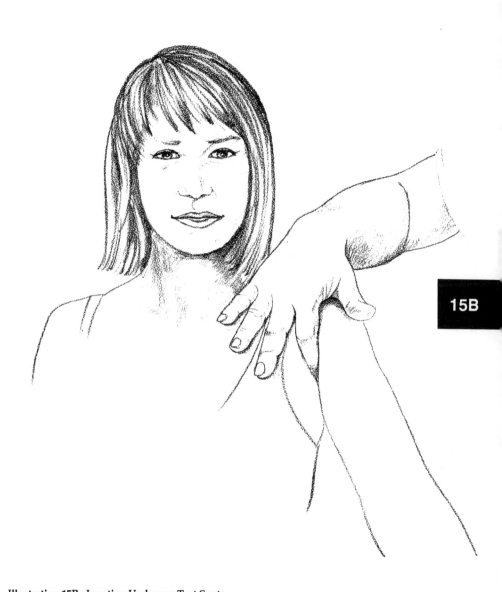

Illustration 15B. Locating Underarm Test Spots.
You can tell if you are touching the Underarm Test Spot properly if your finger is caught in the crease of the armpit when Subject's arm is lowered (pp. 29, 149, 159).

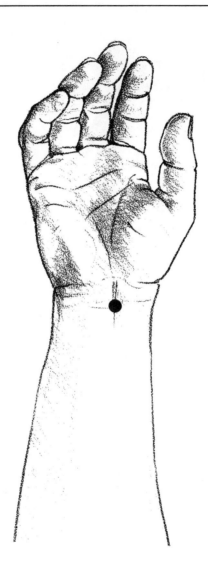

16

Illustration 16. Spots #19 R&L.
Located on center of inside right and left wrist. Used to strengthen indicator muscle if it is weakened by touching Allergy Tap Underarm Test Spots (pp. 29, 149).

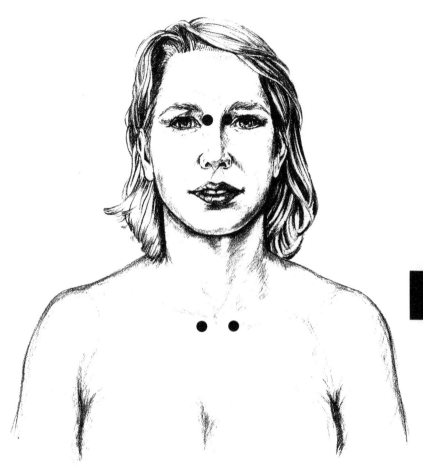

17A

Illustration 17A. Spots #20 R&L.
Located on right and left side of bridge of nose at inner corner of eye.

Spots #22 R&L.
Located on chest at junction of collarbone, first rib, and breastbone, on right and left side.

Both these sets of spots are used as Tapping Spots in Allergy Tap and Tolerance Tap procedures (pp. 34, 46, 47, 150, 155, 156, 159, 161).

17BC

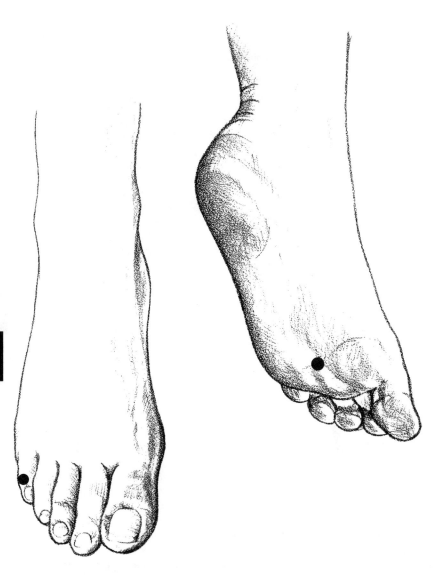

Illustration 17B. Spots #21 R&L.
Located on outer edge of right and left little toe, just below nail. Used in Allergy Tap and Tolerance Tap (pp. 34, 46, 47, 150, 155, 156, 159, 161).

Illustration 17C. Spots #23 R&L.
Located in the center of the ball of the foot. Used in Allergy Tap and Tolerance Tap (pp. 34, 46, 47, 150, 155, 156, 159, 161).

Tolerance Testing
& Tolerance Tap

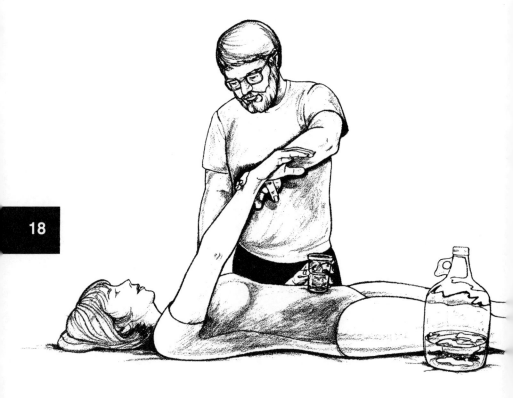

Illustration 18. Tolerance Testing, Lying Position.
Position of Tester and Subject, with test substance in container on Substance Placement Area. For Tolerance Testing, Subject or Tester next touches Tolerance Test Spot while Tester tests indicator muscle (pp. 43, 44, 152, 153).

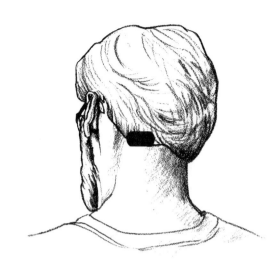

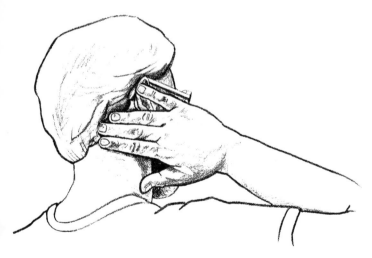

19AB

Illustration 19A. Tolerance Test Spots, #24 R&L.
Located on right and left side of back of neck. Only one spot needs to be touched.
Used for Tolerance Testing (pp. 43, 152).

Illustration 19B. Locating Tolerance Test Spot.
To be sure you are touching Tolerance Test Spot, lightly place fingertips on soft spot
just under skull on one side of back of neck (pp. 43, 152).

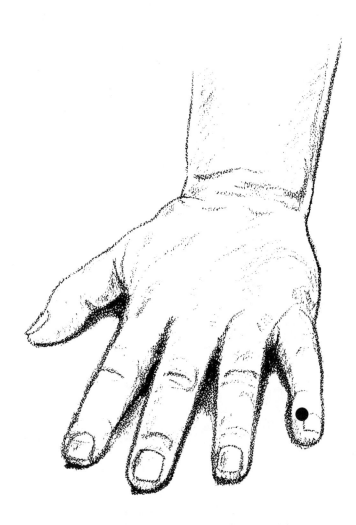

20A

Illustration 20A. Tolerance Test Spot Strengthening Points, #25 R&L.
Located on inside edge of right and left little finger, at base of nail. Used to strengthen indicator muscle if it is weakened by simply touching Tolerance Test Spot (pp. 44, 153, 160).

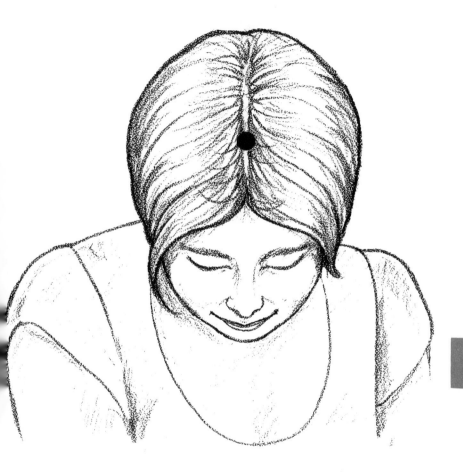

20B

Illustration 20B. Spot #10.
Located on top of head, at point reached by middle finger when palm is placed on bridge of nose. See Illustrations 8B and 8C for locating this spot. Used here for strengthening indicator muscle when it is weakened by touching Tolerance Test Spot. Also used for Special Balancing Procedure, as indicated in Illustration 8A (pp. 44, 153, 160).

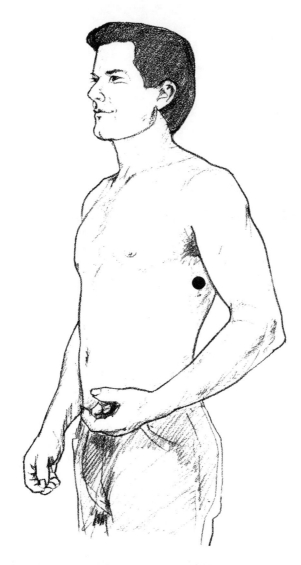

21A

Illustration 21A. Tolerance Tap Test Spots, #4 R&L.
Located on right and left sides, halfway between crook of elbow and armpit. Also used for Balancing Tap, Allergy Tap and Tolerance Tap, as indicated in Illustration 5C (pp. 45, 154, 160).

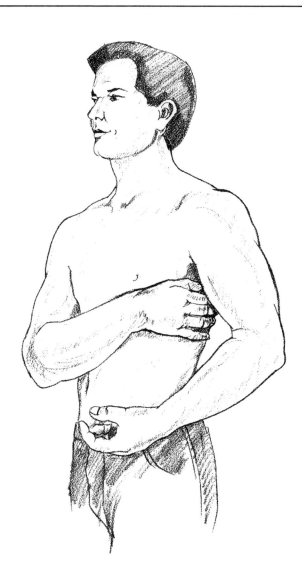

21B

Illustration 21B. Holding Tolerance Tap Test Spot.
Subject is holding one Tolerance Tap Test Spot. Tester would hold the other one (pp. 45, 154, 160).

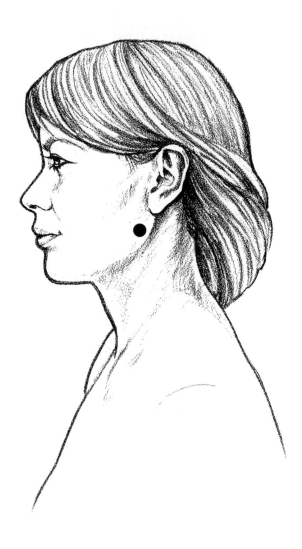

22A

Illustration 22A. Spots #26 R&L.
Located at corner of right and left jaw. Used to strengthen indicator muscle if it is weakened simply by touching Tolerance Tap Test Spots (pp. 45, 154).

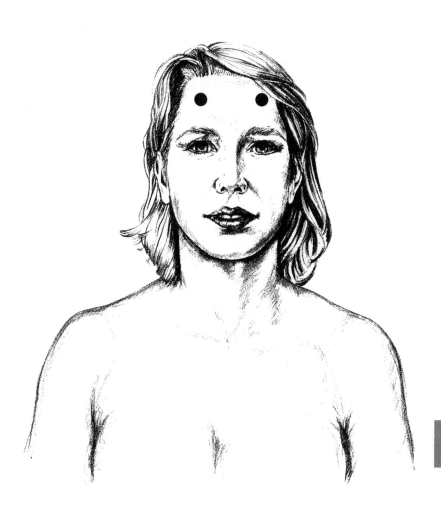

Illustration 22B. Spots #27 R&L.
Located on forehead, above center of right and left eye, at bottom edge of frontal eminence. Used to strengthen indicator muscle if it tests weak on simply touching Tolerance Tap Test Spots (pp. 45, 154).

22B

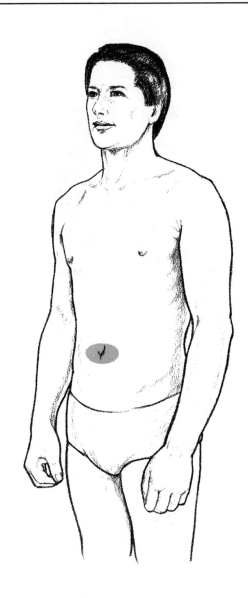

23A

Illustration 23A. Tolerance Area A, Area #28.
Navel area. Note that test substance is placed over Substance Placement Area, *below* navel. Used in Tolerance Tap procedure (pp. 46, 155, 161).

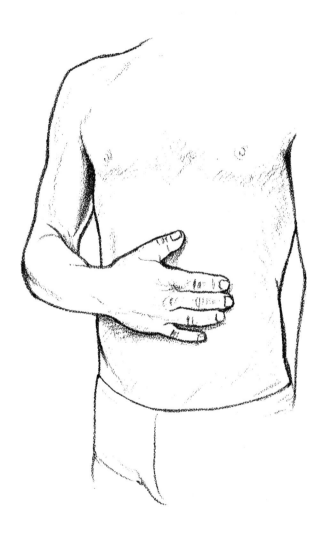

23B

Illustration 23B. Holding Tolerance Area A.
Subject places palm over Tolerance Area A. This area contains many reflex points for the body's energy system (pp. 46, 155, 161).

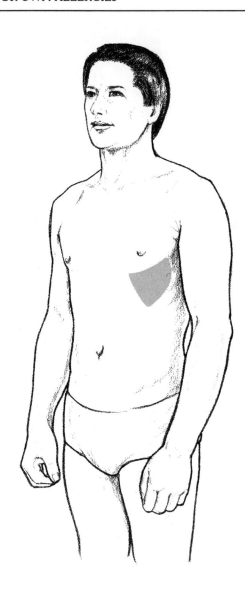

24A

Illustration 24A. Tolerance Area B, Area #29.
Located over left rib cage. Used in Tolerance Tap procedure (pp. 47, 156, 161).

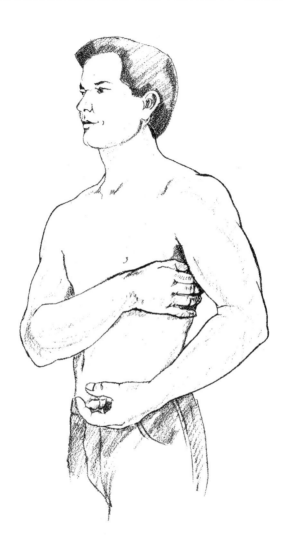

24B

Illustration 24B. Holding Tolerance Area B.
The hand is placed over left rib cage, with little finger along bottom of ribs, fingers spread slightly. Either hand may be used, as long as the same area is covered (pp. 47, 156, 161).

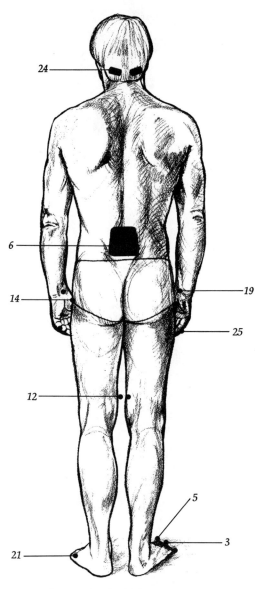

Illustration 25A. Summary of Spots 1-29, Back View.
For detailed descriptions of these spots, refer to the individual Illustrations in this section.

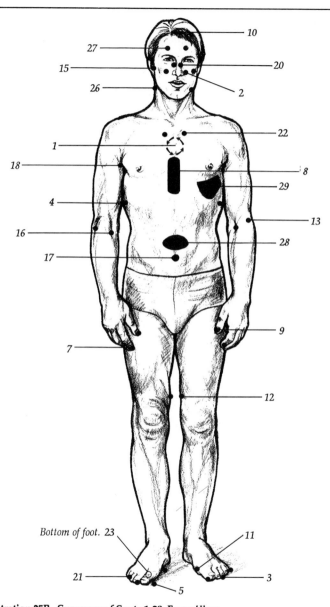

Bottom of foot. 23

Illustration 25B. Summary of Spots 1-29, Front View.
For detailed descriptions of these spots, refer to the individual Illustrations in this section.

25B

APPENDICES

Appendix A

Complete Procedures

Be sure to read through the entire set of instructions before you begin. By understanding the complete process you will achieve better results.

Although these instructions may seem overwhelming at first glance, if you follow each step carefully in turn they will work just as depicted.

All illustrations mentioned in these instructions will be found in the special Illustrations section, preceding the Appendices. The Illustrations pages have dark index bars along the edges for easy reference.

Once you learn the general procedures then you may find that Appendix B, with its shortened instructions, will be easier to follow, since it presents only the essential steps, leaving out less commonly needed variations.

CAUTION: **Remember that in the course of following the instructions in this book, you may be exposed to substances to which you are highly reactive. If you know or suspect that you have severe sensitivities to certain substances, use extreme caution in handling them. If in any doubt whatsoever about how to deal with such substances, consult a properly qualified professional.**

I. MUSCLE TESTING

In order to determine whether you are allergic to a substance you will need to know how to do muscle testing. The reasoning behind muscle testing is discussed in Chapter 2; however, all you need to do here is follow the instructions.

The following simple procedure for muscle testing requires two people. The person administering the test is called the Tester and the person being tested is called the Subject.

Before doing any muscle testing it is a good idea for both the Tester and the Subject to do the following simple energy balancing process, the *Balancing Tap*. This will help insure that the testing works in the most sensitive and repeatable manner.

A. Balancing Tap

The collarbones meet the sternum (breastbone) to form a V shape at the base of the neck. The Energy Balancing Spot (EBS, or area 1), is located on the sternum about 2 inches below this V; there usually is a small bump on the breastbone where the second ribs attach to the sternum (see Illustration 1 in Illustrations section). Imagine a 3-inch diameter circle centered around the EBS (1 1/2 inch radius from the center of the spot). Going in a counterclockwise direction (as the Tester views the Subject), tap around the circle several times for about 30 seconds (perhaps 100 taps, using one or two fingers, as shown in Illustration 1). Tap firmly but gently and be careful with the fingernails. Pretend you are tapping an eggshell as hard as you can without breaking it. Some people are more sensitive than eggshells, so ask if it hurts; if so, tap more gently. You may tap either yourself or the other person. This procedure is called the Balancing Tap.

B. Muscle Testing

Now for the method:

1.The Subject stands in a relaxed position with the feet slightly apart; be comfortable and balanced. The Subject then holds out one arm, palm down, about 45 degrees off to the side and about 45 degrees up (see Illustration 2A). Either arm may be used. (Note: The exact position of the arm isn't critical, but you should become accustomed to doing muscle testing in a consistent way so that you can develop a sense of how the muscles feel as they are being tested. Different muscles will feel different as they are being tested.)

2. The Tester stands facing the Subject, and places one hand on one of the Subject's shoulders (for balance) and the other on the Subject's opposite forearm, slightly above the wrist, so that the Tester can press down on the extended arm. Be sure the Subject's elbow is kept straight. Rather than pressing with the palm the Tester can use all four fingers, or may only need to use one or two fingers to exert the necessary pressure, depending on the Subject's strength (see Illustrations 3A and 3B). The Tester says "Hold," waiting a moment to allow the Subject to comply, and then presses down on Subject's arm, smoothly and steadily increasing the pressure for a period of 2-4 seconds, up to about 8-10 pounds of pressure for most people. If the "indicator muscle" is strong, the Subject will be able to keep the arm raised even with this pressure. If the indicator muscle is weak, the Subject's arm will give way (see Illustration 2B). In this case, both Tester and Subject should repeat the Balancing Tap procedure described above (step IA) before continuing with the testing. If this does not work try the Special Balancing Procedure described in step 4 below. If that still does not work, then perhaps you are pressing too hard, overpowering the muscle rather than testing it. Practice with another person, use less pressure, reread the instructions carefully, or wait until later. Should none of this work, even after repeated attempts, then see Chapter 10 for suggestions about how to find an experienced professional to help out. Sometimes a strong emotional involvement with someone can interfere.

A special note for the Subject: It is important to remember that muscle testing is *not* a test of your strength, your health, or your character. It is a perfectly normal reaction for your muscles to become weak when you are exposed to a substance that interferes with your body's energy. Don't feel that you have to use all your strength to fight the Tester's pressure on your arm. If you are straining, clenching your teeth, or holding your breath you are working at it too hard. Hold firmly without fighting it. Relax and enjoy the experience, and you will learn a great deal about how your body works.

3. If the indicator muscle tests strong, you can now demonstrate muscle testing. Have the Subject say "Yes," and test the muscle simultaneously. The indicator muscle should remain strong on testing. Now have the Subject say "No," again testing at the same time. The muscle should now test weak. This may work better with the Subject's other hand placed over the navel area at the same time. Then broadly but gently pinch the muscle being tested (1 or 2 inches below the top of the shoulder on the side of the arm; see Illustration 4A). The muscle should again test weak. Next "unpinch" the muscle (by moving the fingers apart rather than squeezing as to pinch; be sure to press against the muscle hard enough; see Illustration 4B) and retest. Unpinching is sometimes delicate. If unpinching does not restrengthen the muscle, just have the Subject move the arm around for a few seconds. This time the muscle should be strong. Next, have the Subject say, "My name is . . .," using his or her correct name. The arm muscle should test strong. Now have the Subject say, "My name is . . .," giving a false name. The arm muscle should now test weak. Again, these may work better if the Subject's other hand is placed over the navel. As a final test (and perhaps the most sensitive) have the subject place one palm over the navel and repeat the muscle test. Again, the arm should test strong.

If all four of these test procedures produce the results described, the arm muscle is properly indicating and you can go on to do the allergy testing.

4. If you do not obtain the proper muscle response on the tests in step 3, perform the following Special Energy Balancing procedure.

a.i. Tap spots **2R** & **2L** (right and left cheekbone, just below the center of eye), **3R** & **3L** (outer edge of right and left second toe, just below the nail), **4R** & **4L** (on the right and left side, at level halfway between crook of elbow and armpit), **5R** & **5L** (inner edge of right and left big toe, just below the nail; see Illustrations 5A, B, and C). Then:

a.ii.Touch lightly and continuously each of the following for about 30 seconds: Area 6 (mid-lower back at belt level) simultaneously with spots 7R & 7L (inside edge, toward thumb, of right and left index finger at base of nail; see Illustrations 6A and 6B), and then area 8 (along center of breastbone) simultaneously with spots 9R & 9L (side of thumb away from fingers, at base of nail; see Illustrations 7A and 7B).

a.iii.Touch lightly and hold for about 30 seconds, as above, spot 10 (top of skull, at end of middle finger when palm is placed on bridge of nose; see Illustrations 8A, B, and C).

b.i.Then do this special muscle test:
Using either of Subject's arms, do the regular muscle test as above. Then, testing the Subject's same arm, Tester uses the other hand. For example, if for the regular muscle test the Subject's left arm is used for testing, then ordinarily the Tester's right hand is used to press the Subject's arm. Now Tester switches hands and tests the Subject's left arm with Tester's left hand. It takes longer to describe it than to do it! If the same arm tests strong using each hand, then go on to step 5. If the same arm tests weak using one hand and strong with the other hand, then also do the next Special Balancing procedure.

b.ii.Touch lightly and hold for about 30 seconds spots 11L & 12L simultaneously, and 11R & 12R simultaneously (see Illustrations 9A and 9B); or 13L & 14L simultaneously, and 13R & 14R simultaneously (see Illustrations 10A and 10B). Spots 11 (inside edge of foot, 1/3 distance between ball of foot and back of heel) and 12 (inside upper leg, 1/4 distance between knee and crotch) are very slightly better but less convenient than spots 13 (just above crook of elbow, outside edge of arm) and 14 (base of thumb, outside edge, center of fleshy part).

The regular Balancing Tap procedure plus this special procedure will be adequate 99.9% of the time. This special procedure will not often need to be used.

5. After performing the Special Energy Balancing procedure (if necessary), go back to step 3 and recheck the test questions. All the responses should now be appropriate.

NOTE: For any testing procedure, the indicator muscle must be properly energy balanced. Be sure to perform at least one of the simple tests in step 3 from time to time during the testing session to make sure that the indicator muscle is still strong and balanced. Don't attempt too much in any one session because the muscle can become fatigued. Depending on the Subject, 15 or 20 minutes should be enough. Excessive testing may cause the muscle to be a bit sore for a couple of days, but otherwise does no harm. Excessive soreness also indicates that too much pressure is being used in testing. Alternate testing the right and left arms occasionally to help avoid fatigue.

C. Muscle Testing in Lying Position

Generally, when you are using muscle testing for allergies, it will be more convenient if the Subject is lying down. The muscle testing procedure in the lying position is essentially the same as for standing, except that the Subject in the lying position holds the arm straight up from the body, at an angle of about 30-60 degrees (less for people with stronger muscles), rather than out to the side (See Illustration 11, and compare with the standing position as shown in Illustrations 2A and 2B). The Tester presses straight down on this extended arm. Testing the arm muscle in this position may not feel exactly the same as when the arm is held off toward the side while standing, so experiment with this position until you are familiar with it.

D. Emotional Reactions Influence Muscle Testing

Sometimes you may get the "wrong" results when you do muscle testing because of the emotional involvement between the Subject and the Tester, or because the Subject (or the Tester) has an unconscious emotional investment in making the test come out "right." For this reason, you may find it difficult to do muscle testing on people with whom you have a strong emotional connection, such as family members, your lover, or your boss. You may find it simpler and more convenient to do this work with a more neutral partner—a neighbor, a friend, or a relative with whom you don't live.

II. ALLERGY TESTING

Now that you know how to do muscle testing, you can go on to test for allergies to specific substances.

A. Test Material

Detailed explanations of how and what to collect for testing are given in Appendix D, but for now simply select some food or other substance to which you think you might be allergic. If you want to test yourself for wheat allergy, you can simply use a slice of bread (but remember that bread contains more than just wheat). If you want to test yourself for milk allergy, put a little milk in a closed container (a glass or cup will work just fine, but is more likely to spill). If you suspect you are allergic to cats, have someone collect some cat hair and place it in a plastic bag or small jar. It doesn't matter whether the substance being tested is in a sealed container or open to the air; if you are allergic to it the test will work either way. The closed container, however, will reduce your exposure to the substance and help prevent allergic reactions if you are strongly allergic.

B. Test Procedure

As explained under Muscle Testing, you will need to do this allergy test with someone else. The person administering the test is the Tester, and the person being tested is the Subject.

1.The Subject may be standing, sitting, or lying down. However, as we have explained above, the lying position is most convenient. In order for allergy testing to be accurate, the indicator muscle in the arm must be strong to begin with. If it is not, it must be properly balanced, using the Balancing Tap described in the section on Muscle Testing above.

2. Touch one of the Allergy Test Spots (spot **15R** or **15L**; see Illustrations 12A and 12B) just in front of the ear, on either the right *or* the left side. (Either the Tester or the Subject can touch this spot, but for the sake of simplicity let us assume the Subject touches this spot on the opposite side from the arm being used for muscle testing, using his other arm.) This Test Spot should be touched only while the muscle testing is actually being performed, so as not to fatigue the reflex. Just touch it lightly; there is no need to exert pressure.

Now, while the Subject is touching the Allergy Test Spot with one hand (and before the substance is placed on the Substance Placement Area described below), the Tester tests the Subject's arm as described under Muscle Testing, to make sure that the indicator muscle is reacting properly "in the clear." The muscle should test strong.

Note: A very small proportion of people will test weak on simply touching the Allergy Test Spot. If this should happen to you, the muscle can usually be strengthened by using the following procedure:

a. Gently tap the Allergy Test Spots (spots **15R** & **15L**) with the fingertips, on BOTH the right and the left sides (either one at a time or simultaneously). These spots should be tapped for about 30 seconds, about 90 times.

b. Tap the Muscle Strengthening Spots (spot **16R** & **16L**; see Illustration 13) just above the crease of the elbow, on both the right and left upper arm, in the same manner as described above.

If you follow these procedures and the indicator muscle still tests weak when Subject touches the Allergy Test Spot, discontinue testing for the time being. Wait until another day, or repeat the testing with another person as Tester; perhaps there is an emotional interchange going on which is interfering with the testing procedure. If the problem persists, see Chapter 10 to find help.

Now that the indicator muscle tests strong, proceed to the next step.

3. Expose the Subject to the test substance as follows: Place the test substance (in a container or by itself) on the Subject's abdomen, just below the navel, about two inches. We will refer to this loca-

tion as the Substance Placement Area (area 17; see Illustration 14A). If the Subject is lying down, the substance can just be placed on the abdomen; if the Subject is sitting or standing, either person can hold it in place, or it can be tucked under the Subject's belt or waistband (see Illustration 14B).

4. With the Subject touching the Allergy Test Spot, and with the test substance in position on the Substance Placement Area, test the Subject's arm again. If the muscle now tests *weak*, the Subject is *allergic* to the substance being tested. If the muscle now tests *strong*, the Subject is *not allergic* to the test substance. By repeating the procedure a couple of times in the beginning you can assure yourself that this process really does work. Now you may go on to try another substance.

Once you have identified a substance to which the Subject is allergic, you can then proceed to the Allergy Tap method described below and in Chapter 3. But first, you will need to determine whether the Allergy Tap will work for this particular substance.

III. ALLERGY ENERGY BALANCING

A. Will the Allergy Tap Correction Work for This Person and This Substance?

To determine whether you are in the 90 percent who can be helped by the Allergy Tap method (see Chapter 2), follow the procedure described below. In actual practice, once you have learned the Allergy Test procedure (as described in Chapter 1), you should immediately follow the test procedure for a particular substance with the Allergy Tap Test, to determine whether the Allergy Tap procedure will work in this case. With a given person the Allergy Tap might work for one substance but not another. It might also work at another time if not now.

1. Make sure that the indicator muscle in the Subject's arm is strong; if necessary, balance the muscle as described in the section on Muscle Testing above.

2. Subject and Tester now lightly touch the Allergy Tap Underarm Test Spots, (spots **18R** & **18L**, in the armpit) as shown in Illustrations 15A and 15B. Make sure that both Underarm Test Spots are touched, one by the Tester and the other by the Subject. These spots should be touched, with light pressure, only during the actual muscle testing. If the indicator muscle tests strong in the clear (touching the underarm points but without exposure to the test substance), continue on with step 3.

If the indicator muscle is weak, strengthen it with the following procedure:

a. Lightly touch (simultaneously) spots **19R** & **19L** (center of inside of wrist) for 30 seconds (see Illustration 16).

b. Retest. The muscle should now be strong. If not, wait until another time or seek other help as described in Chapter 10.

3. As in the Allergy Test method described in the section above, expose the person to the test substance by placing it over the Substance Placement Area (area **17**) on the Subject's abdomen just below the navel. Tester tests the Subject's arm muscle while the Underarm Test Spots (spots **18R** & **18L**) are being touched; see Illustrations 15A and 15B. If the muscle tests *weak* on exposure, the Allergy Tap *will work* for this person and this substance. If the muscle tests *strong*, the Allergy Tap *will not work* at this time to eliminate the Subject's allergy to the test substance. If future attempts also indicate that the Allergy Tap method will not work, it may be necessary to use the SET method, performed by a qualified professional (see Chapter 10).

B. *The Allergy Tap Procedure*

Once you have identified a substance to which the Subject is allergic, and for which the Allergy Tap will work, you can proceed to perform the Allergy Tap procedure to eliminate the Subject's allergy to that substance. While it doesn't matter whether the Subject is sitting, standing, or lying down for this procedure, it will usually be easier if the Subject is lying down. Since the treatment involves touching spots on the feet, the Subject's shoes, and preferably socks, must be removed.

1. Expose the Subject to the test substance. This time the exposure to the substance can be enhanced, though it may not be necessary. Instead of simply placing the substance in a closed container on the Substance Placement Area below the navel, the Subject can actually place a little of the substance in his or her mouth, if it is a food; sniff it, if it is a perfume or some other inhaled substance; touch it, if it is a chemical or cosmetic; etc. However, if the Subject is known or suspected to be extremely allergic to the test substance, *be careful*, and keep the substance in a closed container while the Allergy Tap method is administered. You can then repeat the procedure later, if needed, with enhanced exposure to the substance, although this usually is unnecessary.

2. Now, while the Subject is being exposed to the substance as described above, eight sets of Tapping Spots are lightly tapped with the fingertips. It doesn't matter who taps the spots, or in what order. One possible arrangement will be described in detail, but you can vary it as you choose, as long as all spots are tapped on both the right and left sides. Each set of Tapping Spots (right and left) should be tapped lightly for 30 seconds, about 35 times. Both sides may be tapped simultaneously. Spots 20, 21, 22, and 23 (each, right and left) may be tapped in any combination and any order, as may Spots 2, 3, 4, and 5 (each, right and left; these latter spots were also used for balancing, earlier).

(a) Gently tap spots **20R** & **20L** (left and right side of the nose, at the inner corner of the eye; be careful of the eye). Then tap spots **21R** & **21L** (on the outer edge of each little toe just below the nail). These spots are shown in Illustrations 17A and 17B.

(b) Tap spots **22R** & **22L** (on the chest, left and right sides of the breastbone at the junction of the first rib and the collarbone). Then tap spots **23R** & **23L** (in the center of the ball of the foot, on the right and left sole). (See Illustrations 17A and 17C).

(c) Gently tap spots **2R** & **2L** (on the cheekbones just below the center of the right and left eye). Then tap spots **3R** & **3L** (on the outer edge of the right and left second toe, just below the nail). (See Illustrations 5A and 5B).

(d) Tap spots **4R** & **4L** (on the right and left sides at the level halfway between the crease of the elbow, when the arm is bent, and the armpit. By crossing the arms and tapping opposite sides, Subject can tap both these points; see Illustration 5C.) Meanwhile, tap spots **5R** & **5L** (on the inner edge of the right and left big toe, just below the nail; see Illustration 5B).

This completes the Allergy Tap procedure. You may now retest for allergy and see that the Subject tests strong.

C. Retesting for Allergy

Repeat the Allergy Test Procedure described above, using the same substance for which you just did the Allergy Tap procedure.

1. If the Subject now muscle tests strong when exposed to the Test Substance, the allergy has been eliminated. If you have been limiting the Subject's exposure to the substance up to this point (i.e., if the substance has been enclosed in a container), you may now want to repeat the allergy test with a stronger exposure to the substance. Remember, the person's tolerance might be low even though the allergy itself has been corrected. If necessary you should repeat the Allergy Tap procedure with the more direct exposure (again: be careful!), but this is rarely needed. You may prefer to wait a few days before continuing because often changes continue to take place for some time after the Allergy Tap is applied.

2. If the Subject tests weak when exposed to the test substance, you may not have tapped the Tapping Spots adequately, or you may have done the Allergy Tap Test incorrectly. Test the indicator muscle *without* exposure to the test substance. If it tests weak, rebalance it before proceeding. Now repeat the Allergy Tap Test. If the test indicates that the Allergy Tap will work, repeat the Allergy Tap procedure. Again, if you just cannot get this to work correctly, contact a professional as described in Chapter 10.

IV. TOLERANCE TESTING

A. *How to Test Your Tolerance Level*

Just as allergy disturbs your body's energy, so does exposure to a larger amount of a substance than your body can tolerate. (However, intolerances disturb different "circuits" in your body's energy system than do allergies.) The difference between allergy and tolerance is discussed in detail in Chapter 4. You can use muscle testing to determine your *tolerance level* for a given substance, and then (in some cases) increase your tolerance through these energy techniques.

When you used muscle testing to test for allergy, it didn't matter how much of the test substance was used. In testing for tolerance, the amount of the substance is critical, since that is what is being tested. In the case of foods, a convenient amount to begin with is an average serving size. For example, if you are testing the Subject's tolerance for eggs, you could start by exposing the person to one egg. If you are testing tolerance for wheat, you might start with a tablespoon of wheat flour. For many substances, it will be helpful to use a small glass dish or other container, so that you can readily vary the amount being tested. (See Illustration 18.)

1. Make sure that the indicator muscle tests strong. If necessary, do energy balancing as described above. The Subject may be sitting, standing, or lying down, as for allergy testing. However, if an open container is used to hold the test substance it will be more convenient for the Subject to lie down (see Illustration 18).

2. Lightly touch one of the Tolerance Test Spots (spots **24R** or **24L**, at the soft spot just under the skull on either side of the back of the neck; see Illustrations 19A and 19B). It is not necessary to touch both spots simultaneously. As with allergy testing, do not touch the Tolerance Test Spot continuously, but only while muscle testing is being performed, in order not to fatigue the reflexes.

While touching the Tolerance Test Spot (without exposure to a test substance), test the strength of the indicator muscle by testing the Subject's arm. The arm should test strong.

In rare cases, the arm will test weak. To strengthen the arm muscle do the following procedure:

a.Tap for 30 seconds (about 35 times) the Tolerance Test Spot Strengthening Point (spot **25R**) on the inside edge of the right little finger at the base of the nail, while simultaneously touching spot **10** on the top of the head (see Illustrations 20A and 20B).

b.Repeat for the Subject's left little finger (spot **25L** + spot **10**).

c.Retest to make sure the arm now tests strong. If it does not, discontinue testing for the time being. If this situation persists, follow the suggestions in Chapter 10 to find a helpful professional.

Once you have obtained a strong muscle test, proceed to the next step.

3.Place the selected amount of the test substance (either in a container or by itself) on the Substance Placement Area (spot **17**), on the abdomen just below the navel (Illustration 14A). This testing position is shown in Illustration 18.

4.While the Tolerance Test Spot is being touched and the test substance is in place on the abdomen, the Tester tests the Subject's arm.

a.If the muscle tests *strong*, the Subject's *tolerance is greater* than the sample amount. In this case, *increase* the sample size and repeat the test until you determine the amount just slightly less than is required to weaken the indicator muscle. This is the *tolerance level*.

b.If the arm tests *weak*, the amount is already *above the Subject's tolerance level*. Reduce the amount of test substance and repeat the muscle testing until you find the level at which the arm tests strong. This is the *tolerance level*.

Common sense will suggest how to increase or decrease the amount of the test substance. If the arm tests strong with one egg, try two eggs, then three. Obviously, there is little point in testing the Subject for six dozen eggs, since no one is likely to eat that many eggs at one time. To reduce the amount of egg, you may need to break the egg and separate out part of it, say a half. Or you can boil the egg and cut it in half, in thirds, or fourths. (You do not need to determine the tolerance level in order to increase tolerance, but you will not know how much tolerance increase has been achieved unless you do so.)

B. Can the Tolerance Level Be Increased, for This Person and This Substance?

The next test procedure will determine whether the Tolerance Tap procedure can be used to increase the Subject's tolerance for the substance in question.

1. Make sure that the indicator muscle is strong, rebalancing it if necessary. Then, with the Subject lying down, touch both Tolerance Tap Test Spots, on the right and left sides at a level halfway between the crook of the elbow (when the arm is bent) and the armpit (spots **4R & 4L**, Illustrations 21A and 21B; used previously for balancing and for allergy). The Subject may place one hand over the Tolerance Tap Test Spot on the same side as the arm being used for muscle testing, while the Tester places one hand over the Test Spot on the side opposite the arm being tested. The Tester then tests the Subject's free arm. If this test (without exposure to any substance) is strong, then go on to step 2 below. If the muscle tests weak to begin with, strengthen it first by doing the following:

a. Touch and hold for about 30 seconds spots **26L & 27L** simultaneously. Then:

b. Touch and hold spots **26R & 27R** simultaneously. Spots 26RL are located at the corner of the jaw; spots 27RL are located on the forehead, straight above the center of the eye and on the bottom edge of the "frontal eminence"— the small ridge running across the forehead about an inch and a half above the eyebrows (see Illustrations 22A and 22B).

If for some reason you cannot use the Tolerance Tap Test Spots on the sides, there are also Test Spots on the inner edge of the right and left big toe, just below the nail (spots **5R & 5L**; see Illustration 5B). These Test

Spots are not quite as effective as those on the sides, however, and are not as easy to use.

2. Expose the Subject to any amount of the substance, and test the muscle as described above. If the arm muscle tests *weak*, the Subject's tolerance for the test substance *can be increased* by the Tolerance Tap method. If it tests *strong*, the Tolerance Tap method *will not work* to increase the Subject's tolerance for this substance, and the longer SET method will need to be done by a qualified professional. When the Allergy Tap method is effective for increasing tolerance, it works about 96 percent as well as the SET method. However, tolerance increase can be obtained in only about 20% of the cases even with the SET method, as explained in Chapter 4.

V. TOLERANCE ENERGY BALANCING

A. Tolerance Tap Procedure

To increase tolerance, where it can be increased with the energy method, do the following:

1. Expose the Subject to any amount of the substance, as described above.

2. Subject then places one palm over the navel area, Tolerance Area A (area 28, Illustrations 23A and 23B).

3. With the Subject's palm over Tolerance Area A and the test substance on the Substance Placement Area (spot 17, Illustration 14A) on the abdomen, tap spots 20 through 23 (Illustrations 17A, B, and C), right and left sides, as described below. Tapping is continued for 30 seconds, about 35 times, for each set of spots. Any combination of spots 20 through 23 may be tapped individually or simultaneously.

(a) Gently tap spots **20R & 20L** (on both the left and the right side of the bridge of the nose, at the inner corner of the eye; see Illustration 17A). Be careful to do this gently, so as not to injure the eye.

(b) Tap spots **21R** & **21L** (on the outer edge of the right and left little toes, just below the nail; see Illustration 17B).

(c) Tap spots **22R** & **22L** (on both the left and right side of the breastbone at the junction of the collarbone and the first rib; see Illustration 17A).

(d) Tap spots **23R** & **23L** (in the center of the ball of the foot, on the right and left sole; see Illustration 17C).

4. Now the Subject places the right hand over Tolerance Area B (area **29**, Illustrations 24A and 24B), placing the hand over the left rib cage with the little finger along the bottom of the ribs and the fingers spread slightly. (It's OK to use the left hand, also, but be sure that the same area on the left side is covered, whichever hand is used.) With Subject covering Tolerance Area B and the test substance (any amount) on the Substance Placement Area (spot **17**), tap spots 2-5 (Illustrations 5A, B, and C), right and left sides, as follows. Each spot is tapped gently for 30 seconds, about 35 times. Any combination of spots 5-8 may be tapped simultaneously.

(a) Gently tap spots **2R** & **2L** (on the cheekbones just below the center of the right and left eye; be careful not to injure the eye. See Illustration 5A).

(b) Tap spots **3R** & **3L** (on the outer edge of the right and left second toe, just below the nail; see Illustration 5B).

(c) Tap spots **4R** & **4L** (on the right and left sides at a level halfway between the crease of the elbow, arm bent, and the armpit; see Illustration 5C).

(d) Tap spots **5R** & **5L** (on the inner edge of the right and left big toe, just below the nail; see Illustration 5B).

Note that all *Tapping* Spots are the same for Allergy Tap and Tolerance Tap procedures. The only difference is that for the Tolerance Tap the Subject places his hand over the Tolerance Areas, A or B, while the tapping is done.

You may now proceed to retest the Subject's tolerance level for the test substance.

B. Retesting Tolerance Level

Make sure the indicator muscle is still strong and rebalance if necessary. Using an amount of the test substance just larger than the previously determined tolerance level, repeat the tolerance test as described above. If the indicator muscle now tests strong for this amount, increase the test amount until the new tolerance level is determined. Generally, tolerance can be increased by two to six times the original level through use of this Tolerance Tap method.

Appendix B

Short Version of Procedure with Flowchart

[NOTE: Numbers in brackets refer to sections of Appendix A.]

MUSCLE TESTING

1. **Balancing Tap:** Tap Energy Balancing Spot (center of breastbone, Illustration 1) about 100 times, 30 seconds [IA].

2. Test Subject's arm muscle [IB1-2]. If strong, go to step 3. If weak, redo step 1, or go to Appendix A, IB4.

3. Test Subject's arm muscle while Subject says Yes, No; gives true name and false name; and while pinching and unpinching arm muscle [IB3]. If indicator muscle responds appropriately, go on to Allergy Testing. If responses are not appropriate, go to Appendix A, IB4.

ALLERGY TESTING

4. Make sure indicator muscle is strong (see Muscle Testing, above).

5. Touch Allergy Test Spot in front of right or left ear (Illustrations 12A&B) while testing Subject's arm muscle [IIB2].

If strong, go on to step 6.
If weak, go to Appendix A, IIB2a-b.

6. Place test substance on Substance Placement Area on Subject's abdomen (Illustrations 14A&B), while simultaneously touching Allergy Test Spot and testing indicator muscle.
   If muscle is weak, Subject is allergic to the test substance.
   If strong, Subject is not allergic to the substance [IIB3-4].

ALLERGY TAP

7. Make sure indicator muscle is strong; if necessary, rebalance as described under Muscle Testing, above.

8. Touch Allergy Tap Underarm Test Spots (Illustrations 15A&B), while testing indicator muscle in arm [IIIA2].
   If strong, go on to step 9.
   If weak, correct with Appendix A, steps IIIA2a-b.

9. **Allergy Tap Test:** Place test substance on Substance Placement Area on Subject's abdomen (Illustrations 14A&B). Test indicator muscle while Underarm Test Spots are being touched [IIIA3]. If weak, the Allergy Tap will work; proceed to step 10. If strong, Allergy Tap will not work; repeat testing for another substance, or discontinue.

10. **Allergy Tap:** While exposing Subject to test substance (using enhanced exposure if appropriate), tap Tapping Spots 20-23 R&L, and 2-5 R&L, as follows:
    20: beside nose at inner corner of eye (Illus. 17A).
    21: outer edge little toe, just below nail (Illus. 17B).
    22: chest, junction of collarbone, first rib, and breastbone (Illus. 17A).
    23: center of ball of foot (Illus. 17C).
    2: cheekbone, below center of eye (Illus. 5A).
    3: outer edge 2nd toe, just below nail (Illus. 5B).
    4: side, halfway between crook of elbow and armpit
       (Illus. 5C).
    5: inner edge big toe, just below nail (Illus. 5B).
    Spots 20-23 may be tapped in any combination simultaneously, as may Spots 2-5 [IIIB1, 2a-d].

11. Retest for allergy by repeating step 6, above. If Subject now tests strong, the allergy has been eliminated. If weak, repeat tapping as in step 10, or check indicator muscle as in step 7 [IIIC1-2].

TOLERANCE TESTING

12. Make sure indicator muscle is strong; if necessary, rebalance as described under Muscle Testing.

13. Touch Tolerance Test Spot at back of Subject's neck (Illustrations 20A&B) while simultaneously testing indicator muscle in Subject's arm [IVA2]. If arm tests strong, go on to step 14. If weak, go to Appendix A, steps IVA2a-c, to correct.

14. Place selected amount of test substance on Substance Placement Area on Subject's abdomen. While Tolerance Test Spot is being touched, test indicator muscle. If strong, tolerance is greater than the sample amount; increase sample size until muscle tests weak to find tolerance level. If muscle tests weak, tolerance is less than sample amount; reduce amount of test substance until muscle tests strong. This is the tolerance level [IVA4a].

TOLERANCE TAP

15. Make sure indicator muscle is strong; if necessary, rebalance as described under Muscle Testing.

16. Touch Tolerance Tap Test Spots on left and right sides, halfway between crook of elbow and armpit (Illustrations 21A&B), and test the indicator muscle [IVB1]. If arm tests strong, go on to step 17. If weak, go to Appendix A, step IVB1a to correct.

17. **Tolerance Tap Test:** Now place test substance (any amount) on Substance Placement Area on abdomen. Touch Tolerance Tap Test Spots, right and left, while simultaneously testing the indicator muscle in the arm. If weak, tolerance can be increased by Tolerance Tap; proceed to steps 18 and 19. If strong, tolerance cannot be increased by Tolerance Tap; discontinue or try another substance [IVB2].

18. **Tolerance Tap:** Place any amount of substance on Subject's Substance Placement Area. With Subject's palm over Tolerance Area A (navel area, Illustrations 23A&B), tap Tapping Spots 20-23, right and left, as follows [VA1-3]:

    20: beside nose at inner corner of eye (Illus. 17A).
    21: outer edge little toe, just below nail (Illus. 17B).
    22: chest, junction of collarbone, first rib, and breastbone (Illus. 17A).
    23: center of ball of foot (Illus. 17C).

19. Continue with substance on Substance Placement Area. With Subject's hand over Tolerance Area B (left rib cage, Illustration 24A), tap Tapping Spots 2-5, right and left, as follows [VA4]:

    2: cheekbone, below center of eye (Illus. 5A).
    3: outer edge second toe, just below nail (Illus. 5B).
    4: side, halfway between crook of elbow and armpit (Illus. 5C).
    5: inner edge big toe, just below nail (Illus. 5B).

20. Repeat Step 14 to retest tolerance level [VB].

Part 1

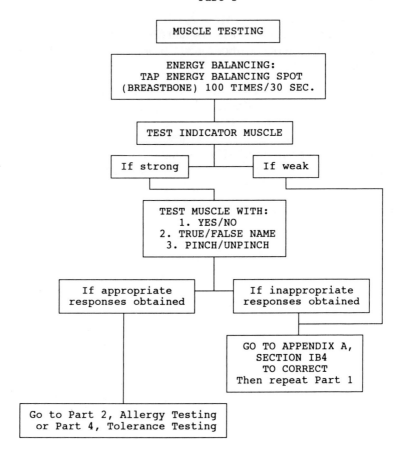

Part 2

```
┌─────────────────────┐
│   ALLERGY TESTING   │
└─────────────────────┘
┌─────────────────────────┐
│ TOUCH ALLERGY TEST SPOT │
│    (IN FRONT OF EAR)    │
│ & TEST INDICATOR MUSCLE │
│       "IN CLEAR"        │
└─────────────────────────┘
```

┌─────────────┐   ┌─────────────┐
│ If strong │   │   If weak   │
└─────────────┘   └─────────────┘

```
┌─────────────────────────┐
│  PLACE TEST SUBSTANCE   │
│     ON SPA (ABDOMEN);   │
│  TOUCH ALLERGY TEST SPOT│
│ & TEST INDICATOR MUSCLE │
└─────────────────────────┘
```

┌─────────────┐   ┌─────────────┐
│ If strong │   │   If weak   │
└─────────────┘   └─────────────┘

```
                        ┌─────────────────────────┐
                        │  GO TO APPENDIX A,      │
                        │     SEC. IIB2a-b        │
                        │      TO CORRECT         │
                        │  Then repeat step 2     │
                        └─────────────────────────┘
```

```
┌─────────────────────────────┐   ┌─────────────────────────┐
│   Subject is not allergic   │   │  Subject is allergic    │
│     to test substance.      │   │    to test substance.   │
│ Repeat with another substance│  └─────────────────────────┘
│      or discontinue.        │
└─────────────────────────────┘
```

```
                        ┌─────────────────────────┐
                        │  Try another substance  │
                        │           or            │
                        │      Go to Part 3,      │
                        │ Allergy Energy Balancing│
                        └─────────────────────────┘
```

Part 3

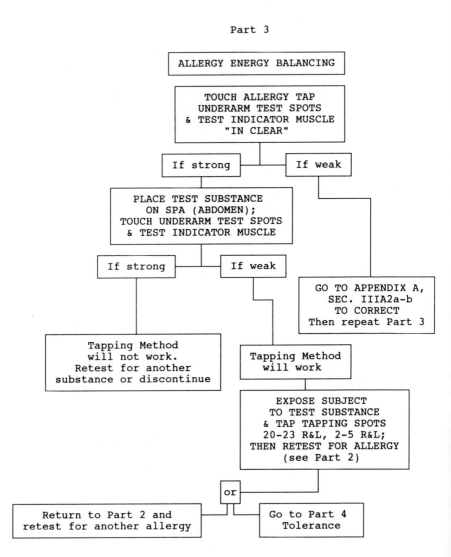

Part 4

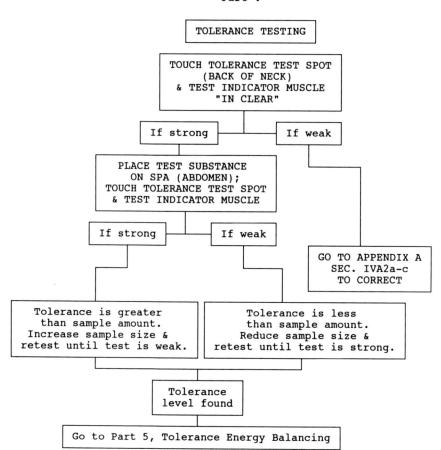

TOLERANCE TESTING

TOUCH TOLERANCE TEST SPOT
(BACK OF NECK)
& TEST INDICATOR MUSCLE
"IN CLEAR"

If strong — If weak

PLACE TEST SUBSTANCE
ON SPA (ABDOMEN);
TOUCH TOLERANCE TEST SPOT
& TEST INDICATOR MUSCLE

If strong — If weak

GO TO APPENDIX A
SEC. IVA2a-c
TO CORRECT

Tolerance is greater
than sample amount.
Increase sample size &
retest until test is weak.

Tolerance is less
than sample amount.
Reduce sample size &
retest until test is strong.

Tolerance
level found

Go to Part 5, Tolerance Energy Balancing

Part 5

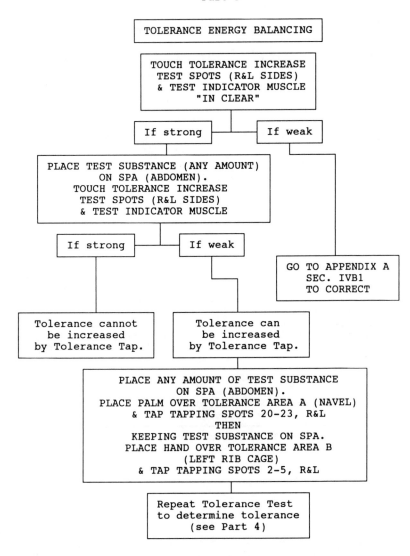

TOLERANCE ENERGY BALANCING

TOUCH TOLERANCE INCREASE
TEST SPOTS (R&L SIDES)
& TEST INDICATOR MUSCLE
"IN CLEAR"

If strong — If weak

PLACE TEST SUBSTANCE (ANY AMOUNT)
ON SPA (ABDOMEN).
TOUCH TOLERANCE INCREASE
TEST SPOTS (R&L SIDES)
& TEST INDICATOR MUSCLE

If strong — If weak

GO TO APPENDIX A
SEC. IVB1
TO CORRECT

Tolerance cannot
be increased
by Tolerance Tap.

Tolerance can
be increased
by Tolerance Tap.

PLACE ANY AMOUNT OF TEST SUBSTANCE
ON SPA (ABDOMEN).
PLACE PALM OVER TOLERANCE AREA A (NAVEL)
& TAP TAPPING SPOTS 20-23, R&L
THEN
KEEPING TEST SUBSTANCE ON SPA.
PLACE HAND OVER TOLERANCE AREA B
(LEFT RIB CAGE)
& TAP TAPPING SPOTS 2-5, R&L

Repeat Tolerance Test
to determine tolerance
(see Part 4)

Appendix C

Location of Reflex Points

Spot	Location	Illus.	Actual Name
#1 Energy Balancing Spot	Breastbone, 2 inches below "v" at bottom of neck	1	Thymus
#2RL	Cheekbones, just below center of each eye	5A	St 1
#3RL	Outer edge of second toe, just below the nail	5B	St 45
#4RL Tolerance Increase Spot	On side, at level halfway between crease of elbow and armpit	5C	Sp 21
#5RL	Inner edge of big toe, just below the nail	5B	Sp 1
#6	Mid lower back, at belt level	6A	Li NL

#7RL	Index finger, base of nail, side toward thumb	6B	Li 1
#8	Along center of breastbone	7A	Lu NL
#9RL	On thumb, base of nail, away from fingers	7B	Lu 11
#10	On top of skull, at end of middle finger when palm is placed on bridge of nose	8A	H NV
#11RL	Inside edge of foot, 1/3 of distance between ball of foot and back of heel	9A	Sp 4
#12RL	Inside upper leg, 1/4 distance between knee and crotch	9B	Sp 10
#13RL	Just above crease of elbow, outside edge of arm	10A	Lu 5
#14RL	Base of thumb, outside edge, center of fleshy part	10B	Lu 10
#15RL Allergy Test Spot	In front of ear	12A	Tw 21
#16RL Muscle Strengthening Spot	Just above crease of elbow, upper arm	13	Cx 3

#17 Substance Placement Area	On abdomen, just below the navel	14A	Cv 6
#18RL Underarm Test Spots	Armpit	15A	H 1
#19RL	Wrist, inside, center	16	Cx 7
#20RL	Beside nose at inner corner of eye	17A	B 1
#21RL	Outer edge of little toe, just below the nail	17B	B 67
#22RL	Breastbone at junction of first rib and collarbone	17A	K 27
#23RL	Center of ball of foot	17C	K 1
#24RL Tolerance Test Spots	Back of neck, to the side of midline	19A	Atlas- Axis Jct.
#25RL	Inside edge of little finger, base of nail	20A	H 9
#26RL	On the cheek at the corner of the jaw	22A	St NV
#27RL	On the forehead, above the center of the eye, on the bottom edge of the "frontal eminence"—the ridge running across the forehead about 1 1/2 inches above the eyebrows	22B	Cv NV

| #28 Tolerance Area A | Navel area | 23A | B & K NV |
| #29 Tolerance Area B | Left side, from bottom of rib cage spreading upward to breast area | 24A | St & Sp NV |

Abbreviations used in this chart:

R   Right side of body
L   Left side of body
NV Neurovascular Reflex
NL Neurolymphatic Reflex

St Stomach Meridian
Sp Spleen Meridian
Li Large Intestine Meridian
Lu Lung Meridian
H   Heart Meridian
Tw Triple Warmer Meridian
Cx Circulation Sex Meridian or Heart Constrictor Meridian
Cv Central Meridian or Conception Vessel
B   Bladder Meridian
K   Kidney Meridian

The numbers beside the Meridian names refer to acupuncture points.

Appendix D

How To Collect Samples For Testing

Collecting and Handling Samples

It is extremely important to be as thorough as possible in your testing of various substances—that is, if you want the maximum benefit from your efforts. In this section you will learn more about how and what to collect for testing. The only general rule is that *anything* with which you might come into contact is something to be concerned about. Unfortunately, a great many of these substances are hidden from our view, and may not have any smell or taste. We must learn how and where to find them.

How you collect the sample depends on the nature of the material. Some items, like an orange or an apple, are easy to test by themselves, but other substances will need to be put in containers, such as plastic sandwich bags,[a] small jars, or bottles. Put about a spoonful of each food or other substance in separate containers. Be sure to label any items that you may later have difficulty identifying.

---

[a] Be sure to test the empty plastic bag, too.

When it comes time to do the actual testing, do not wear any perfumes, fragrances or other cosmetics that might interfere with your reactions. For the same reason, avoid wearing synthetic fabrics, if possible.

With any substance that you collect for testing, be careful to avoid over-exposure. If you suspect that you are quite allergic to something, **be very careful when you collect the sample, or get someone else to collect it for you.** The same cautions apply for the correction procedures. You can use your samples in the same form as for testing, but as we explained in Chapter 3, when you do the correction procedures it is sometimes helpful to enhance your exposure to the substance. For foods, rather than putting the food on the Substance Placement Area on the abdomen, you should put a little right in your mouth, unless you are very allergic to it. In that case do the correction first with the substance placed on the abdomen in a closed container. Retest for allergy, and put the substance in your mouth for further correction only when your sensitivity has been reduced. Test, however, because you may not need any further correction.

Record Keeping

Be systematic. Write down everything you have tested (see sample record form in Appendix F). For items such as molds or fungus, be sure to make a note about where the sample was obtained so that you won't duplicate your efforts later. You might also find it beneficial to write down anything you can even *think* of testing. It could take some time to track down and collect all the items, and you wouldn't want to forget any of them in the meantime.

We have arranged our suggestions for sample collection under categories below, not so much to tell you what to collect as to call your attention to some items you might overlook.

Foods

Foods that should be tested include easily preserved items such as grains, nuts, seeds; beans, peas and other legumes; cooking herbs and herb teas; spices; dried fruits; dry soup mixes; dried dairy products; beverages including coffee and tea. Fresh and perishable foods include fruits, vegetables, meats, seafood, eggs, poultry, dairy products, oils, condiments such as mayonnaise, mustard, vinegar, and packaged foods.

Test a convenient amount of each food. A whole orange or a tomato is easy to handle, but a whole watermelon would be rather awkward. You only need to use a small amount of each item. Again, be sure to label anything about which there might be any doubt.

Try to keep your food test items as simple as possible. When ingredients are combined it is much more difficult to determine what is responsible for an allergic reaction. A casserole containing 15 ingredients may taste wonderful and be nutritious, and it may include something to which you are allergic; but is it only one of the ingredients or all fifteen?

It is best to test things in the form in which you eat them, or might eat them. If something tests OK raw, it will usually be OK cooked. The reverse is slightly less likely, as cooking may destroy some component substance present in the raw form.

Water

One very important item which is easy to overlook for testing is the water you drink, cook with, and bathe in. Collect samples of tap water, distilled water, spring water, well water, and bottled waters such as mineral waters. As we saw in Chapter 4, it is very important to test all sources of water that you use, especially for tolerance, since your body requires large quantities of water every day—quantities that may exceed your tolerance level for the water that you are actually drinking. Water for drinking (and cooking) must test at least 100 ounces per day, and preferably at least 200 ounces per day, in order to be adequate.

Pollens and Flowers

You can buy small samples of various kinds of bee and flower pollens in health food stores. Try to get as many different kinds as possible, from a wide variety of flowers, especially those that are collected locally. Bee pollens are available in bulk, in tablets, or capsules.

Also, simply collect flowers—from your house, your yard, and around your neighborhood. When you go on walks, just pinch off a flower. It doesn't need to be the freshest or most beautiful one. Don't overlook your neighborhood flower shop. A friendly clerk may save samples of old or unusual flowers for you. Remember that it is probably illegal to pick flowers in parks; but when you take walks down the street or in the woods, collect any flowers you see. You may also go into a flower shop and ask them to keep samples of anything that they are going to throw away. Air dry your flower samples, or simply test them fresh.

Besides common flowers, such as roses, tulips, daffodils, wildflowers, etc., don't forget that trees and shrubs also have pollen. The pollen from different plants is produced at different seasons of the year, and different pollens prevail in different areas of the country. You may need to extend your collecting year round, and you can ask friends and relatives from other areas to send you samples of local flowers and pollens.

Once again, we must caution that if you know you have severe allergies to pollens, be very careful when you collect your samples, or get someone else to do it for you. Seal the samples well inside a plastic bag, and keep your sample sealed during the correction procedure until you are sure that your sensitivity has been reduced.

Dust

Probably the easiest way to collect dust is to vacuum as completely as possible and then to use the bag from the vacuum cleaner. Don't forget the attic, basement, top shelves, and back corners of closets. You certainly can't forget the proverbial "under the bed" dust. The entire dust bag can be placed over the Substance Placement Area for allergy testing and balancing (and tolerance work too, of course). Dust content will vary from season to season and from one area of the country to another. Repeat the tests every three or four months for a year. Have friends and relatives save dust for you. Go ahead, get a reputation for collecting weird things.

Dust will consist of various mites, spores from molds, pollens, fibers from fabrics and rugs, and so on, not to mention just plain dirt. Because of this great variety of content, dust can be used to balance numerous allergies. Not much dust is needed, but as much different dust as possible is desirable.

Molds, Fungus, Mildew

Since it is hard to tell one of these from another they will all be considered together. Most of us like to believe that none of these substances are found in *our* living space. Leave some food out for a few days. Does it get moldy? Great! Save it to use for testing (you can scrape off some of the mold and place it in a small bottle). Go through your house, systematically searching out any damp place. Look around the shower or tub. Scrape particles off of any dark or stained area. Check beneath the sink, where the pipes go through the wall, or behind the toilet bowl. Frost-free refrigerators have drip trays. Marvelously yukky stuff can grow there, so collect some of it. The dirt in which your potted plants grow is also a favorite place for molds and fungus. Don't forget those plants *outside*, either. Collect not only some small samples of dirt from outside the house, but also check around the foundation, under the house, the garage, any other outbuildings, the garden, and (be careful here) the neighbor's. Remember, only a very small amount of sample is needed. A small fraction of a teaspoonful is sufficient. Tiny amounts from a large number of areas will be the most helpful and effective.

Cosmetics

Collect samples of personal items such as cosmetics, perfumes, lotions, salves, ointments, creams, toothpaste, shampoo, conditioners and rinses, hair coloring, and deodorants. Be sure to include items used by other household members if you are exposed to them. Men do breathe their wives' perfumes!

When you test cosmetics, you may need to do more than simply place them on the Substance Placement Area on the abdomen. Since cosmetics are used on the skin, often you will get a reliable test only if you actually apply some to the skin at the time of doing muscle testing. Be sure to test a sniff of it, too.

Household Items and Substances

It's easy to overlook the things in your environment that you are exposed to routinely every day. Take a careful look around your house, and make sure that you are testing anything whatsoever in your environment.

Collect samples of clothing, representing different kinds of fabric and also different dyes, waterproofing chemicals, mothballs, etc. Jewelry may contain many allergic substances. Collect fiber from furniture, carpets and bedding, and feathers or fiber from pillows. Remember all your cleaning supplies, including soaps, detergents, fabric softeners, bleaches, cleansers, waxes, polishes, oils, rug shampoos, and air refreshers. Collect samples of glues, pastes, household cements, and epoxy resins. Check your basement or tool shed for paints, varnishes, removers, roofing and insulating materials, and gardening supplies including insecticides, herbicides, fertilizers, even lawn-mower fumes. If you have a swimming pool or a spa, collect samples of the chlorine or other chemicals used in it. Don't forget plastic items, including kitchen containers and toys.

Drugs and Medicines

Test any medicines that you are using, including medicinal herbs, vitamins and nutritional supplements, prescription and over-the-counter drugs. Don't forget to include any "recreational" substances that you may use. Go through your medicine cabinet and your first aid supplies and test everything that is put into your body or used externally for medicinal purposes.[b] If you are expecting to have dental work done, ask your dentist for small samples of the materials he might use. If you are going to have something permanently placed in your mouth, you might as well make sure it agrees with you!

---

[b] Don't be surprised or too alarmed if you test allergic or very intolerant to some of your regularly used medicines. You may want to consult with the appropriate health professional about this problem.

Chemicals

You may encounter many different kinds of chemicals in your workplace, your home, or your general environment. Here are suggestions about how to collect some of them.

Be very careful in handling all chemicals because many are highly toxic. Be sure to handle these materials in a well ventilated room or outdoors, and keep your exposure to an absolute minimum. Collect small amounts of gasoline, turpentine, pesticides, paints, solvents, and other substances in carefully labeled bottles. Be sure to follow label instructions when handling these materials, and be aware of any warnings.

To collect smog or auto exhaust, catch it in a bottle. Be sure to seal it tightly.

Matches make good test materials for chemical allergies. Use matches with both white heads and dark heads. Fumes from matches are related to smog since they contain sulfur and phosphorus compounds. Thus matches can be used for correction procedures as well as testing. Strike the match, blow out the flame, and sniff the smoke.

To test yourself for sensitivity to chemicals, be very careful, and try exposing yourself first to the closed container. If exposure to the substance in the closed container is enough to weaken the indicator muscle, then you know it's not OK for you. However, if you test OK with the material in a closed container you may actually need to sniff or touch the chemical for testing. For petroleum chemicals such as gasoline or turpentine, it's reasonably safe to take a tiny sniff. Other chemicals such as pesticides may be much more dangerous. In the case of these substances, you may want to spray or drop a tiny bit on a piece of paper or cardboard, and then take a gentle sniff from the paper. When you do correction procedures with these substances, gently sniff the substance and then put it away in a closed container immediately before you retest, so that you aren't getting further exposure to it.

To prevent the need for prolonged exposure to these chemicals, you can also combine closely related substances and test them simultaneously. Remember that some combinations are dangerous, so when in doubt use them separately. Again, always follow the label instructions when handling chemical materials.

Pets and Other Animals

Everybody knows that cats and dogs have fur to which some people are allergic. But don't forget their saliva. They lick themselves and often people. Hamsters, rabbits, mice, fish, snakes, horses— whatever the pet, don't overlook the possibilities. Remember that horses sweat, cages frequently are layered with wood chips, birds have feathers (check your own feather pillows), and that kitty litter is a mixture of substances.

Although you don't eat your pet's food (or do you?), test it on yourself.[c] Dry food can produce "dust," and any food that has any smell contains substances with which you are coming into contact. Of course, touching the food can result in your absorbing through the skin substances to which you are allergic.

Lastly, keep in mind that neighbors also have pets who might visit (invited or not) and leave a variety of excellent test items.

The Workplace

Take a critical look around the place where you work, and collect samples of everything in your environment that might be causing you problems. Such things as typewriter ribbons, correction fluid, fumes from photocopying machines or blueprint machines, inks, pigments, glues, photographic chemicals and other processing materials should all be tested. In manufacturing facilities, collect samples of any fumes that may be in the air, lubricating materials, and raw materials used in manufacturing. Not everyone works in offices and factories. Gardeners would need to collect fertilizers, pesticides, even the dirt (fungus and mold) to which they are exposed in their work. Artists are exposed to a great variety of often highly toxic substances.

---

[c] See Chapter 5, Surrogate Testing, to learn how to test your pets for allergy and intolerance.

Remember that one element in your workplace is the cosmetics and perfumes that other people may be wearing. Wherever you work, you are also exposed to materials used for cleaning, painting, and maintenance in your environment, and you are probably using the soap provided in the rest room.

The HKPapers™ test extracts (see ordering information in Appendix G) do *not* eliminate the need for collecting the above materials. Although the extracts are very helpful, there is no way to include all the possible things to which you might be exposed. Testing with both your collected materials and the extracts would insure the widest practical coverage of possibilities.

Appendix E

Food Families

The following list of food families will be helpful to you in allergy testing, allergy energy balancing, and tolerance testing and balancing. Many potentially allergic foods are related to other foods, flowers, and herbs, and if you are allergic to one member of such a family you may also be allergic to others. For example, you may discover in allergy testing that you are allergic to potatoes and tomatoes, but you may not realize that tobacco is in the same family, so that you are probably allergic to tobacco also. As another example, beans and peas are in the same family as other less familiar legumes such as clover, alfalfa, and carob. If you are allergic to certain beans or peas, then these other foods are suspect also. When you test allergic to a certain food, it is a good idea to carefully check other foods in the same family; you may find that you are not allergic to them, but it is quite possible that you are.

The same principle applies to tolerance. If you are intolerant of a given food, you are likely to have a low tolerance for related foods and other substances also.

Thus, knowing what foods are in the same family can help prevent tolerance problems. Suppose that you were allergic to wheat, rye, barley, and oats, and that using energy techniques these allergies have now been corrected. You may now have a tolerance for wheat of one cup per week. You may also have a tolerance for rye of one cup, two-thirds of a cup for oats, and one-half cup for barley. This does not mean, however, that you can eat these amounts of *each* food. Especially when foods are related by family, you need to check your tolerance for the family as a whole. You are likely to find that your tolerance for the entire food family combined is a total of one cup per week, rather than one cup for wheat, one for rye, two-thirds for oats, and one-half cup for barley. This table will help to call to your attention food families you should test for when you are checking your tolerances.

Sometimes strong relationships between plants or animals extend beyond family boundaries. For this reason we have grouped certain families together to show that they are related within larger botanical classifications. These groups are called Orders. In the listing below, FAMILY NAMES are shown in all capital letters. Family names *not* separated by blank lines are related to each other, being in the same Order, while the different Orders, while not named, are separated by blank lines. The Orders are not split up across pages. If the relevant food is obvious because of the family name, it is not again specified. For example, the Ginseng Family need not have "ginseng" listed again. The popular family names shown are not always precise, botanically speaking, but are given to help you identify them. Common sources of certain very popular foods are also given, such as tofu (under soy).

We have also listed animal families, and shown how they are related within larger zoological classifications. For example, many people are allergic to seafood. By seeing how the various kinds of seafood are related, such people will have a better idea of which foods they may be sensitive to.

While you may not be able to find giraffe in your local supermarket, if you were a guest at a tribal feast in Africa and knew you were allergic to deer meat, you might want to be wary of the proffered giraffe stew! You will also notice many items which we never ordinarily eat (e.g., poison oak), but which are included to show you how plants or animals are related. Each item is given in the Index, Section 1, as well in the plant family list, Section 2, or the animal family list, Section 3.

SECTION 1

Index To List Of
Plants And Animals

P

Pacific halibut 202
PADDLEFISH FAMILY 202
Palm 194
PAMPANO FAMILY 203
Pansy 198
PAPAYA FAMILY 198
Paradise nut 198
Parsley 199
Parsnip 199
PASSION FRUIT FAMILY 198
Pasta 193
PAWPAW FAMILY 196
Pea 196
Peach 196
Peafowl 204
Peanut 196
Pear 195, 196
Pecan 195
Pennyroyal 199
PEPPER FAMILY 195
PERCH FAMILY 202, 203
Periwinkle 199
Persian melon 200
PERSIMMON FAMILY 199
Peruvian lily 194
Petunia 199
Pheasant 204
PIGEON FAMILY 203
PIG FAMILY 205
Pigweed 195
PIKE FAMILY 202
Pimento 199
PINEAPPLE FAMILY 194
PINE FAMILY 200
Pinenuts 200

Pinto bean 196
Pistachio 197
Plantain 194
Plum 196
Poi 194
Poinsettia 197
Poison ivy 197
Poison oak 197
Poison sumac 197
Polenta 193
Pollack 202
POMEGRANATE FAMILY 198
Pomelo 197
Popcorn 193
Poppy 197
POPPY FAMILY 197
PORGY FAMILY 203
PORPOISE FAMILY 204
POTATO FAMILY 199
Prairie chicken 204
Prairie dog 204
Prickly pear 195
PRIMROSE FAMILY 198
PRONGHORN 205
Prune 196
Puffed rice 193
PUFFER FAMILY 203
Pumpkin 200
Pumpkinseed fish 203
PURSLANE FAMILY 195

Q

QUAIL FAMILY 204
Quince 196
Quinoa 196

Plant Kingdom—Botanical Families

ALGAE, SEAWEEDS
> dulse, kelp (kombu), Irish moss (carrageenan), hiziki, sea palm, sea lettuce, agar, nori, wakame, arame, spirulina, chlorella

GRASS FAMILY
> BAMBOO Subfamily
> GRASS Subfamily
> WHEAT Subfamily
>> wheat, rye, triticale, barley (-bran, -germ, -flour; couscous, gluten, graham, bulgur, malt, breads, pasta, beer, liquors)
> OAT Subfamily
> RICE Subfamily
>> rice (-bran, -polishings, -flour, -syrup, -noodles; puffed rice, rice crackers, rice bread; mochi)
> LEMON GRASS Subfamily
>> lemon grass, citronella
> MILLET Subfamily
> SUGAR CANE Subfamily
>> sorghum, sugar cane (-sugar, -molasses)
> CORN, MAIZE Subfamily
>> corn (-grits, -tortillas, -starch, -bran, -germ, -sweeteners, -oil, -noodles; farina, polenta, hominy, popcorn)

SEDGE FAMILY
> Chinese water chestnuts, chufa (groundnut), sedge

MUSHROOMS
mushroom, truffle

MOLDS
mold, mildew, fungus

YEASTS
baker's yeast, brewer's yeast, torula yeast

COCONUT FAMILY
coconut, sago, date palm

TARO FAMILY
taro (poi), malanga, yautia

PINEAPPLE FAMILY
pineapple

LILY FAMILY
asparagus, onion, chives, leek, shallot, garlic, yucca, African lily, hyacinth, lily, bluebell, aloe vera, tulip
SARSAPARILLA FAMILY
sarsaparilla
YAM FAMILY
yam, yampi
AGAVE FAMILY
agave, mescal, Peruvian lily, narcissus, lily-of-the-field, belladonna lily
IRIS FAMILY
saffron, orris root, gladiolus, iris

BANANA FAMILY
banana, plantain
GINGER FAMILY
cardamom, ginger, turmeric
ARROWROOT FAMILY

ORCHID FAMILY
   orchid, vanilla

PEPPER FAMILY
   black pepper

WALNUT FAMILY
   English walnut, black walnut, butternut, heartnut, pecan, hickory

BEECH FAMILY
   beechnut, chinquapin, chestnut, oak
BIRCH FAMILY
   filbert (hazelnut)

MULBERRY FAMILY
   mulberry, fig, hops, breadfruit, marijuana

MACADAMIA NUT FAMILY

CARNATION FAMILY
   carnation, pink, baby's breath
ICEPLANT FAMILY
   iceplant, New Zealand spinach
AMARANTH FAMILY
   amaranth, cebsia (cockscomb)
CACTUS FAMILY
   prickly pear
PURSLANE FAMILY
   purslane (pigweed)

BUTTERCUP FAMILY
   delphinium, fennel flower, buttercup, anemone (wildflower)

BUCKWHEAT FAMILY
   buckwheat, rhubarb, sorrel
ACEROLA FAMILY
   acerola (Barbados cherry)

SPINACH FAMILY
common beet, sugar beet, Swiss chard, spinach, quinoa, lamb's quarters

PAWPAW FAMILY
pawpaw, custard-apple
MACE FAMILY
true nutmeg, mace
AVOCADO FAMILY
avocado, cinnamon, bay leaf, sassafras
CHINESE LOTUS FAMILY
Chinese lotus

ROSE FAMILY
ROSE Subfamily
hawthorne, blackberry, raspberry, strawberry, boysenberry, logan-
berry, dewberry, longberry, youngberry, rubus, rose
APPLE Subfamily
apple, pear, quince
PEACH Subfamily
peach, plum, prune, almond, apricot, cherry, nectarine, sloe (black-
thorn)
CURRANT FAMILY
hydrangea, currant, gooseberry
LEGUME FAMILY
MIMOSA Subfamily
acacia (mimosa), gum acacia, caro
SOYBEAN Subfamily
licorice, lentil, peanut (-oil, -butter), kidney bean, navy bean, bush
bean, string bean, pinto bean, lima bean, mung bean, tonka bean,
pea, black-eyed pea, chick pea (garbanzo), soybean (-sprouts, -oil,
-grits, -milk, -protein, -sauce; tamari, tofu, miso, tempeh, lecithin,
most natural vitamin E), Windsor bean, broad bean, gum traga-
canth, senna, cassia, indigo, laburnum, sweet pea, gorse, wisteria,
clover, tamarind, alfalfa (-sprouts), fenugreek, jicama, kudzu

MUSTARD FAMILY
>kale, collards, common cabbage, savory cabbage, Brussels sprouts, broccoli, cauliflower, kohlrabi, cardoon, mustard, watercress, turnip, rutabaga, radish, horseradish, mugwort

POPPY FAMILY
>California poppy, common poppy

RUE FAMILY
>CITRUS Subfamily
>>citron, lemon, lime, grapefruit, orange, tangelo, tangerine, pomelo, kumquat

EUPHORBIA FAMILY
>poinsettia, tapioca, rubber tree, cassava, yucca, castor oil plant

GERANIUM FAMILY

IMPATIENS FAMILY

FLAX FAMILY

NASTURTIUM FAMILY

OXALIS FAMILY
>oxalis, carambola

HORSE CHESTNUT FAMILY
>horse chestnut, lychee nut, soapberry

CASHEW FAMILY
>cashew, pistachio, mango, poison oak, poison ivy, poison sumac

MAPLE FAMILY
>maple sugar, syrup

GRAPE FAMILY
>grape, raisin, cream of tartar

CASCARA SAGRADA FAMILY

COTTON FAMILY
hollyhock, okra, althea root, cotton, hibiscus
COCOA FAMILY
gum karaya, cocoa, chocolate, kola
BASSWOOD FAMILY
basswood, linden

CAMELLIA FAMILY
camellia, tea
PAPAYA FAMILY
papaya
KIWI FAMILY
kiwi

DOGWOOD FAMILY
dogwood, cornel

MYRTLE FAMILY
guava, allspice, clove, bottle brush flower, myrtle, eucalyptus
FUCHSIA FAMILY
POMEGRANATE FAMILY
BRAZIL NUT FAMILY
Brazil nut, paradise nut

BEGONIA FAMILY
PASSION FRUIT FAMILY
passion fruit, granadilla
VIOLET FAMILY
violet, pansy
TAMARISK FAMILY
ANNATTO FAMILY

PRIMROSE FAMILY
primrose, cowslip

CARROT FAMILY
  carrot, celery, celeriac root, parsley, parsnip, anise, caraway, dill, chervil, fennel, angelica, sweet cicely, lovage, coriander (cilantro), cumin, gotu kola
GINSENG FAMILY

HEATHER FAMILY
  wintergreen, blueberry, cranberry, huckleberry, bearberry, azalea, rhododendron, heather

PERSIMMON FAMILY
  persimmon, kaki
CHICLE FAMILY
  chicle (chewing gum)

GENTIAN FAMILY
JASMINE FAMILY
  jasmine, lilac, olive
OLEANDER FAMILY
  oleander, periwinkle

POTATO FAMILY
  petunia, potato, tomato, tomatillo, eggplant, tobacco, all red and green peppers (bell, pimento, chili, cayenne, etc.), curry powder
MINT FAMILY
  coleus, mint, basil, lavender, marjoram, rosemary, sage, horehound, savory, oregano, chia, catnip, pennyroyal, balm, thyme, Chinese artichoke, bergamot, clary, dittany, hyssop
MORNING GLORY FAMILY
  morning glory, sweet potato, bindweed
SESAME FAMILY
  sesame (tahini)

VERVAIN FAMILY

SNAPDRAGON FAMILY
snapdragon, foxglove, monkey flower (musk), nemesia
MILKWEED FAMILY

GARDENIA FAMILY
gardenia, coffee
HONEYSUCKLE FAMILY
honeysuckle, elderberry
VALERIAN FAMILY

SQUASH FAMILY
cucumber, zucchini, loofa, gherkin, winter squash, pumpkin, summer squash, muskmelon, honeydew, Persian melon, Spanish melon, watermelon, Crenshaw, cantaloupe

LETTUCE FAMILY
lettuce, endive, chicory, common artichoke, Jerusalem artichoke (sunchoke), sunflower, marigold, aster, chrysanthemum, cape marigold, zinnia, dandelion, chamomile, goldenrod, safflower, floss flower, felicia (marguerite), boneset (comfrey, symphytum), burdock root, escarole, tarragon, coltsfoot, salsify, santolina, yarrow, wormwood, tansy

HOLLY FAMILY
holly, yerba mate

CAPERS FAMILY

HORSETAIL FAMILY
horsetail (shavetail)

CEDAR FAMILY
cedar, ash, juniper (gin), cypress
PINE FAMILY
pine, pine nuts, fir
REDWOOD FAMILY

Animal Kingdom
—Zoological Families

SCALLOP FAMILY

OYSTER FAMILY

COCKLE FAMILY
CLAM FAMILY

ABALONE FAMILY
SNAIL FAMILY
    escargot

SQUID FAMILY

CRUSTACEANS
    SHRIMP FAMILY
    LOBSTER FAMILY
    CRAB FAMILY
        crabs, urchins, caviar (eggs)

INSECTS
    BEE FAMILY

SHARK FAMILY

STURGEON FAMILY
  sturgeon, beluga, caviar (eggs)
PADDLEFISH FAMILY

TARPON FAMILY
HERRING FAMILY
  herring, shad, menhaden, caviar (eggs)
ANCHOVY FAMILY
SALMON FAMILY
  salmon, trout, caviar (eggs)
WHITEFISH FAMILY
SMELT FAMILY
PIKE FAMILY

SUCKERFISH FAMILY
CARP FAMILY
CATFISH FAMILY

EEL FAMILY

COD FAMILY
  cod, haddock, pollack, silver hake

MULLET FAMILY
  mullet, silversides

FLOUNDER
  right eyed flounder, Atlantic halibut, Pacific halibut
SOLE FAMILY

OCEAN PERCH FAMILY
SEA ROBIN FAMILY
  sea robins, sea tags

PUFFER FAMILY

GROUPER FAMILY
   rockfish, striped bass, grouper, white perch
RED SNAPPER FAMILY
GRUNT FAMILY
BASS FAMILY
   bass, sunfish, pumpkinseed, bluegill
PERCH FAMILY
   yellow perch, walleye, pike
BLUEFISH FAMILY
PAMPANO FAMILY
DOLPHIN FISH FAMILY
   mahi mahi
WHITING FAMILY
   weakfish, croaker, whiting, drumfish
PORGY FAMILY
MACKEREL FAMILY
   mackerel, tuna, bonito
BUTTERFISH FAMILY
   butterfish

BULLFROG FAMILY

TURTLES
TERRAPIN FAMILY
SNAKES
ALLIGATOR FAMILY

DUCK FAMILY
   duck, goose, eggs

PIGEON FAMILY

GROUSE FAMILY
    grouse, prairie chicken
QUAIL FAMILY
    quail, peafowl, pheasant, domestic chicken (eggs, -white, -yolk)
GUINEA FAMILY
    guinea fowl
TURKEY FAMILY
    turkey (eggs)

OPOSSUM FAMILY

RABBIT FAMILY
    rabbit, hare

RODENTS
    rats, mice
MUSKRAT FAMILY
WOODCHUCK FAMILY
    red squirrel, woodchuck, prairie dog
BEAVER FAMILY

WHALES
DOLPHIN FAMILY
PORPOISE FAMILY

CANINE FAMILY
    dogs
WOLF FAMILY
BEAR FAMILY
RACCOON FAMILY

FELINE FAMILY
  cats, lion, tiger

SEAL FAMILY
SEA LION FAMILY
WALRUS FAMILY

ELEPHANT FAMILY

HORSE FAMILY

PIG FAMILY
HIPPOPOTAMUS FAMILY
CAMEL FAMILY
  camel, llama
DEER FAMILY
  deer (venison), elk
MOOSE FAMILY
  moose, caribou, reindeer
GIRAFFE FAMILY
PRONGHORN ANTELOPE FAMILY
CATTLE FAMILY
  cattle (cow), Brahman, American bison, African buffalo, sheep, goat
  (milk, cheese, butter, yoghurt, ghee, keifer)

Appendix F

Testing Record Form

The Record Form shown here is just a suggestion. You can photocopy this form for your own use (you will need more pages than are given here), you can use it as a model with your own variations, or you can make up some other form you feel comfortable with. The important factor is that you keep some record of what you discover in your testing.

Place your name on the form, so that different family members won't become confused. Enter the "date" of the testing in the first column. The "item tested" comes next. Separate columns for items which are "OK" or "not OK" are given so that it is easier to see at a glance which is which. Mark the "can correct?" column if the Underarm Test indicates the allergy can be corrected. Likewise, mark the "can increase tolerance?" column if the tolerance can be increased. If you determine the actual tolerance level, that can be shown here, too. After finishing any needed corrections, allergy and tolerance increase, mark the final column, "complete." That way you can quickly see which items still need work. Likewise, if there is no allergy and the tolerance is adequate, you can mark the last column since there is no further work to do.

Another copy of the Form is on page 222, for easier copying.

Name_____

date	item tested	OK?	not OK?	can correct?	can increase tolerance?	com-plete

date	item tested	OK?	not OK?	can correct?	can increase tolerance?	complete

Appendix G

Report Form & Miscellaneous

Please send to Dr. Scott some information regarding your experiences using this book. Please keep in mind that he will be unable to answer each person individually, but that each reply will be tabulated as part of Dr. Scott's research. Continue your comments with additional pages if you wish. Rather than remove these pages, feel free to photocopy the report forms.

(Please Print)   I am ____male ____female.   Age_____

Your Symptom Scores (Chapter 1):

Date: ____   ____   ____   ____

Totals: ____   ____   ____   ____

Prior to using this book were you medically diagnosed with any disease or illness?

When: What:

What other methods of treatment did you use?

How did they work?

What changes occurred after using the methods described in this book?

Do you attribute these changes to what you learned with this book?

HOW TO ORDER OTHER MATERIALS

If the order form on the last page of this book is already gone, feel free to photocopy this and the next page.

Please let me know when the following become available:

☐ *Cure Your Own Allergies in Minutes: the VIDEO.*

☐ *Energy, Allergy, and Your Health.* Second edition.
    A companion to *Cure Your Own Allergies in Minutes.*

☐ *Relieve your Own Emotional Distress and Phobias in Minutes.*

☐ *Dr. Scott's High-Calorie Weight Control Diet*
    (and Program for Good Health).

☐ *Improve Your Own Intellectual Functioning and Creativity in Minutes.*

☐ *Emotions Training.*

☐ HKPapers™ (other than *Candida albicans*).

Send your orders or requests for information to:

Health Kinesiology Publications
1032 Irving Street, Suite 340
San Francisco, Ca 94122
USA
(415) 566-4611

order form over:

ORDER FORM

Please send me:

☐ ____ copies of *Cure Your Own Allergies in Minutes*
US$14.95 plus **$2.50** shipping and handling
(total: **$17.45**) (plus **$0.90** tax in California).

$_____

☐ ____ HKPapers™ for *Candida albicans*.
US$3.50 including shipping, handling, and tax.

$_____

☐ Quantity discount information.

Total: $_____

Please print or type:

name _____

address _____

_____

city _____ state _____ zip _____

telephone (_____) _____ - _____

Send your check or money order in U.S. or equivalent Canadian funds to:

Health Kinesiology Publications
1032 Irving Street, Suite 340
San Francisco, Ca 94122
USA

Jimmy Scott, Ph.D.

Dr. Scott received his Ph.D. in Physiological Psychology from the University of North Carolina in 1966. His academic experience includes research at the National Institute of Mental Health and positions at three University medical schools. He has published numerous research papers in scientific and medical journals.

Beginning an independent practice in 1973 led to his development of new and powerful concepts in Holistic Health, especially after learning kinesiology a few years later. Combining nutritional knowledge with the techniques of kinesiology allowed Dr. Scott to determine very precisely and specifically for each individual exactly what nutrients were needed, which supplements were best to use, and which foods to eat or to avoid. The allergy concepts, as described in this book, were subsequently developed. Health, however, involves much more than nutrition and allergy, so Dr. Scott set about to develop analogous methods in all the areas relevant to health. These other areas are discussed in forthcoming books, some of which have already been mentioned in this volume. Although the nutrition and allergy work is very important to many people, Dr. Scott's work in developing the energy techniques in psychological applications is truly revolutionary, allowing dramatic changes in behavior to take place quite rapidly and easily.

In addition to his very busy practice, Dr. Scott also writes magazine articles on health topics, appears frequently on radio and TV, and travels throughout the world lecturing and teaching seminars on Health Kinesiology to other professionals.

Kathleen Goss, M.A. is a writer in the interrelated fields of health and consciousness. She is co-author (with Michael Weiner, Ph.D.) of *Maximum Immunity* (Houghton Mifflin, 1986), *Nutrition Against Aging* (Bantam, 1983), *The Art of Feeding Children Well* (Warner, 1982) and *The Complete Book of Homeopathy* (Bantam, 1982), and contributed as writer and editor to works by Jack Schwarz, Ken Dychtwald, Arthur Young, and others. She is the former Managing Editor of *Applied Psi Newsletter,* and has written on a wide range of subjects including nutrition, herbal medicine, executive health, healing, aging, and appropriate technology. She is the author of two volumes of poetry, and is presently writing a novel that incorporates concepts of energy healing.

Claudia Ricketts Wagar is an artist who has been in the San Francisco Bay area for some 15 years. Illustrating and designing for major advertising and publishing firms, she has a spectrum of styles. Her work has been well received in a wide variety of markets.

This Book has had a complex evolution. It began with Kathy transcribing tapes of some of my lecture material and some of our discussions (on CP/M computer #1, using the WordStar word processing program). This would end up on my computer (CP/M computer #2, using NewWord, a WordStar compatible word processing program) and on paper for our further discussion and my changes. Often this cycle would repeat several times until we "got it right." In the midst of all this I switched to computer #3 (MS-DOS compatible with the WordPerfect word processing program). I used computer #2 to convert the disks from computer #1 to a format readable by computer #3. WordPerfect then had to convert the WordStar format into its own format in order to continue. At the very end Kathy switched to computer #4 (MS-DOS compatible, with WordPerfect). Initial paper copies were with a dot-matrix printer, with later versions done on a letter-quality printer. The final version, with very few hand-done additions or changes, was made ready for the book printer—"typeset"—with a laser printer.

Everyone knows that computers save paper. I estimate that some 7500 sheets of paper were used to get these final pages ready! I would guess that had the "old fashioned" method of paper and pen or typewriter been used then the paper consumption would have been more like a thousand pages. On the other hand, the speed with which computers allow us to make changes in our work is so beneficial that a few thousand pieces of paper is a trivial price to pay. I cannot imagine working any other way, now.

Index

Record Form

Name_____

date	item tested	OK?	not OK?	can correct?	can increase tolerance?	com-plete

HOW TO ORDER OTHER MATERIALS

Rather than remove this order form, feel free to photocopy this and the next page.

Please let me know when the following become available:

☐ *Cure Your Own Allergies in Minutes: the VIDEO.*

☐ *Energy, Allergy, and Your Health.* Second edition.
　　A companion to *Cure Your Own Allergies in Minutes.*

☐ *Relieve your Own Emotional Distress and Phobias in Minutes.*

☐ *Dr. Scott's High-Calorie Weight Control Diet*
　　(and Program for Good Health).

☐ *Improve Your Own Intellectual Functioning and Creativity in Minutes.*

☐ *Emotions Training.*

☐ HKPapers™ (other than *Candida albicans*).

Send your orders or requests for information to:

Health Kinesiology Publications
1032 Irving Street, Suite 340
San Francisco, Ca 94122
USA
(415) 566-4611

order form over:

ORDER FORM

Please send me:

☐ ____ copies of *Cure Your Own Allergies in Minutes*
    US$14.95 plus **$2.50** shipping and handling
    (total: **$17.45**) (plus **$0.90** tax in California).

                                                    $_____

☐ ____ HKPapers™ for *Candida albicans*.
    US$3.50 including shipping, handling, and tax.

                                                    $_____

☐ Quantity discount information.

                                    Total: $_____

Please print or type:

name _____

address _____

_____

city _____ state _____ zip _____

telephone (_____) _____ - _____

Send your check or money order in U.S. or equivalent Canadian funds to:

Health Kinesiology Publications
1032 Irving Street, Suite 340
San Francisco, Ca 94122
USA